Advance Praise

"Not your usual herbal remedy book, this is a treasure of inspiration for bringing healing foods to the table. I expect it to become splattered with sauces and imprinted with buttery fingers as all well-loved cookbooks are."

—*Chris Dalziel*, founder of Joybilee Farm

"Devon makes it easy to incorporate medicinal herbs into everyday life with her delightful recipes. Using herbs can feel daunting, but her straightforward approach is accessible to everyone."

—*Stacy Karen*, founder of No Fuss Natural

"If you believe as I do that food is the key to our health, the pages of this book are delicious confirmation. I am looking forward to cooking recipes from this innovative new book!"

—*Janet Garman*, author and founder of Timber Creek Farm

"Devon has a knack for inspiring us to think outside the box and use healing herbs in our everyday cooking. The recipes are sure to inspire creativity in the seasoned herbalist and give confidence to those just beginning their herbal journey."

—*Angi Schneider*, founder of SchneiderPeeps

"Devon Young's wealth of knowledge is evident in the thoughtful combination of ingredients, and the recipes are completely drool-worthy. This book is a very digestible way to include herbalism in daily life, and a tasty one!"

—*Stephanie Rose*, award-winning author and founder of Garden Therapy®

"This book takes the mystery out of an herbalist's kitchen. What a tasty way to make food your medicine."

—*Connie Meyer*, founder of Urban Overalls

"Devon has a style that makes things attainable for all home herbalists and cooks, from beginners to more advanced. This book will be a go-to in our home for years to come."

—*Emily Maze*, founder of This Crazy Maze

"*The Herbalist's Healing Kitchen* is the perfect introduction for those interested in expanding their knowledge of wellness while utilizing their larders and backyard offerings. It's simple yet thoughtful, practical with just a touch of whimsy, and beautifully and lovingly written. Devon Young is a woman who knows her material, and her desire to inspire others is evident in every page."

—*Rhea Hoeflok*, founder of Hedgerow Cottage

"Another must-have book by Devon Young. Who knew some of the things I enjoy weekly have the power to help my body thrive! Can't wait to give these mealtime herbal recipes a go!"

—*Hannah "Suzie" Nicole*, founder of Muddy Oak Hen House

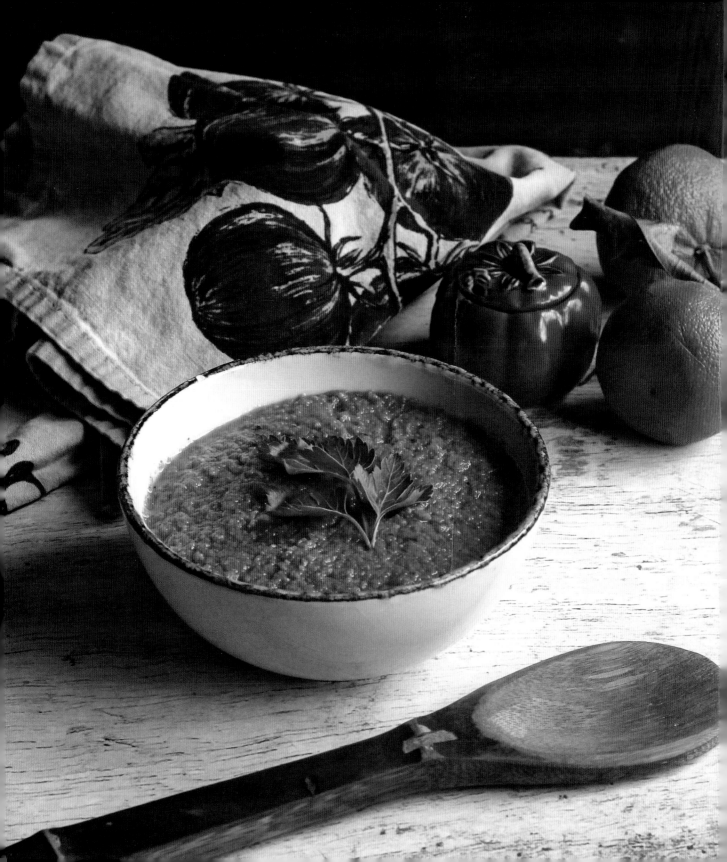

THE HERBALIST'S
HEALING KITCHEN

Use the Power of Food to Cook Your Way to Better Health

DEVON YOUNG

Author of *The Backyard*
Herbal Apothecary and Founder of
Nitty Gritty Life

PAGE STREET
PUBLISHING CO.

First published in 2019 by
Page Street Publishing Co.
27 Congress Street, Suite 105
Salem, MA 01970
www.pagestreetpublishing.com

Distributed by Macmillan, sales in Canada by The Canadian Manda Group.

23   22   21   20   19   1   2   3   4   5

ISBN-13: 978-1-62414-997-9
ISBN-10: 1-62414-997-9

Library of Congress Control Number: 2019939664

Cover and book design by Kylie Alexander for Page Street Publishing Co.
Photography by Devon Young

Printed and bound in China

DEDICATION

Thank you to my family. You are the most critical and amazing taste-testers a home cook could have!

TABLE OF CONTENTS

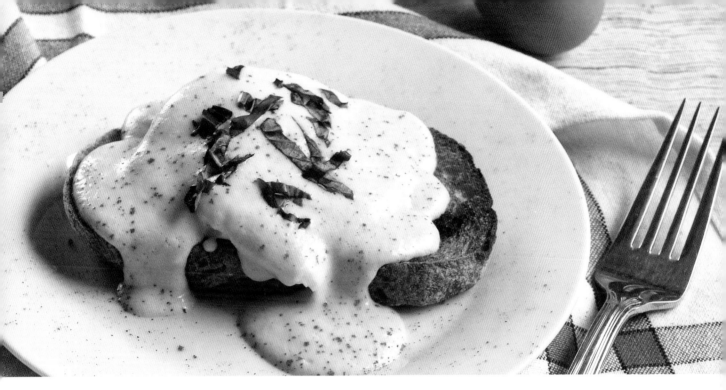

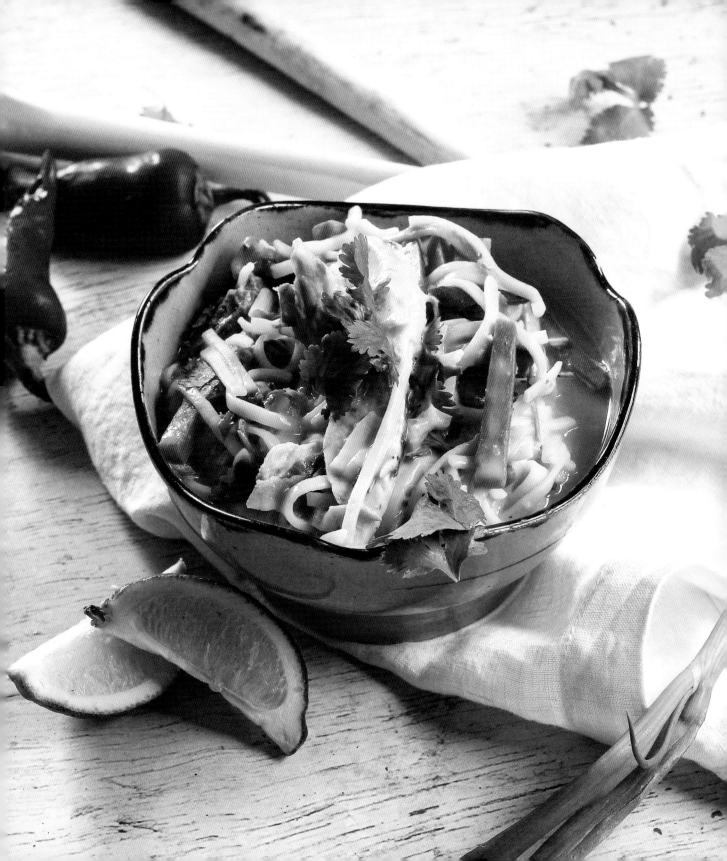

FOREWORD

The title of Devon Young's new book is appropriate, because herbalists do indeed have healing kitchens! Most of us use our kitchens as command central: after we contemplate the many complexities of how to best approach our health and the health of those we love, it's in our kitchens that we whip up an herbal preparation or design a healthy, wholesome meal. *The Herbalist's Healing Kitchen* shows us what it looks like to create foods with intention—the intention to make better, to make well and to support our body's ability to balance and heal.

Devon makes the point that paying attention to your body is key to addressing its needs. She recalls instinctively knowing that the peppermint candies offered at restaurants as an after-dinner sweet were soothing to her stomach, but it was only in hindsight that she made the connection between the consumption of peppermint and the relief she felt. Food can have an immediate or a delayed effect on us, but the point is to take notice. Does a specific food help you feel better, give you more energy, help you think more clearly, make you sleepy or perhaps make you feel anxious? Once we begin to notice the more obvious manifestations of the food we are eating, we can tune in to the more subtle expressions. When we start to listen to our bodies, we gain insights that allow us to choose foods that are right and good for us.

I've made my way around quite a few kitchens as a caterer, traveler, mother of three and herbalist, and I've learned a few culinary tricks here and there. I know how to use a wide variety of ingredients to make healthy, delicious and sometimes even inspiring recipes. But when Devon shares that flavor is the secret language of food, revealing to us the action of that food, I had to stop and think for a moment. Yes, indeed, flavor is the informer advising our taste buds, but also much more importantly, other body systems. The question is, how many of us use that information to our advantage? Understanding flavors such as sour, pungent, bitter, salty and sweet provides us with an entirely new set of tools with which we can guide our culinary and herbal repertoire.

The one thing we all can do is to choose what we put into our bodies. We can make good, informed choices, as Devon does in *The Herbalist's Healing Kitchen*. Whether we feel the need to recharge and restore, boost our immune system, build cardiovascular health, jump-start our reproductive system or ease a troubled mind, we can design recipes using ideal foods and herbs that fit our particular needs. Your salivary glands may be working overtime as you read through these mouthwatering and original recipes that are both purposeful and delicious! Lemon Congee with Poached Eggs & Radish Microgreens (page 38), Chai-Spiced Crème Brûlée (page 110) and Coconut Rice Pudding with Cardamom & Rose (page 113) are just a few to look forward to. You're in for a real treat!

—Marlene Adelmann
Herbalist and Founder of the Herbal Academy

INTRODUCTION

For me . . . it all really started with food.

When I was growing up, herbs and spices weren't used medicinally in our home—but they were most certainly used in our cooking. My father fostered my love of epicurean wonders through his fragrant herb garden and his penchant for watching cooking shows. I learned early on in life how rosemary brings levity to a rich leg of lamb and how the peppery kick of watercress pairs beautifully with citrus and seafood. I observed how the red-and-white mints offered with the check at the end of a restaurant meal could soothe a troubled tummy.

I was learning that food is medicine. But I wasn't listening yet.

So quickly we dismiss these valuable lessons. We forget to pay mind to cues the body gives to us. We find ourselves thinking that cures and good health only come with a white coat and a prescription pad, or from shelves of supplements and quick-fix remedies. The more clinical the remedy, the less we relate to it—and the more "effective" it becomes in the collective mind.

We seem to be looking for heroic cures, for instant gratification. And that can only come in a bottle, right? Because, how could the living world really give us everything we need? How could plants, animals, fungi and even tiny microbes offer the key to healthful living? How could we each hold the answers to our own wellness?

Perhaps it is a quirk of human nature. We often strive for the unattainable and yearn for the exotic.

In my work as an herbalist, I see this tendency far too often. People attach themselves to concepts and products, and they place their bets on the latest fads. Everybody is looking for healing in all the wrong places.

True healing begins in the most fundamental of origins. It starts in the food that we eat.

Without proper nourishment, we are building a house on a crumbling foundation. With wholesome, nutritious foods, we fortify our minds and bodies. We build strength. We grow. We perform. We birth. And we heal.

There is a complexity in healing that so often gets overlooked. We reach for the "quick fixes," and we forget how to set the stage for real healing. Healing exists when we are present with each and every choice—and when those choices are made in the interest of good health.

We can create recipes that address a multitude of minor and major health complaints. Simply by making informed food decisions, and by using sub-therapeutic levels of traditional medicinal herbs and spices, we can care for ourselves! We aren't taking gigantic, heroic steps. Rather we are setting ourselves up for true health and healing—the type that lasts.

Food and herbs can coax the mind and body back into a healthy, neutral position. They can open our sinuses, ease an upset stomach and fortify our reserves after a long haul. Common herbs, such as black pepper, rosemary and even parsley, have profound medicinal benefits. Simple foods—ones in your home *right now*—offer nourishment and contain powerful nutrients that promote good health. They can even put a stop to many of our frequent, bodily complaints.

When you learn the medicinal potential in your own kitchen, you can create meals that are deeply healing.

The Herbalist's Healing Kitchen is a guide to choosing and preparing the right foods and herbs to support optimal health. You will learn the everyday foods, herbs and spices that can effectively neutralize conditions—from the common cold to a flatlined libido. You will find detoxifying recipes, fortifying recipes, recipes to improve your cardiovascular system, recipes to promote immunity, recipes to encourage digestion, recipes to make you strong and recipes that deliver sexual and reproductive health.

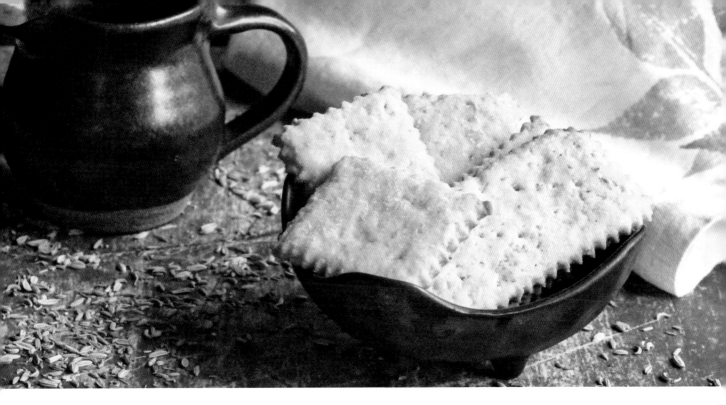

I am going to teach you to identify foods and herbs for their medicinal value and nourishing health benefits. You will come to see your pantry, refrigerator and even the grocery store in a whole new light—one where your daily food choices become customized medicine for your mind and body.

You will learn how to identify the major flavor profiles—sour, pungent, bitter, sweet and salty. And you will learn how these flavors influence the healing actions of foods and herbs. With this knowledge, you can venture beyond the many recipes in this book to turn your kitchen into a healing apothecary.

Let's cast aside the notion that healing comes only with a prescription. Healing starts at home, in our kitchens, with food made by our own hands. Let's discover the kitchen as our source of healing.

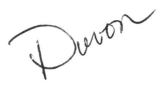

HOW FOODS HEAL

We need food. It satiates our hunger. It fills our stomachs. It meets our nutritional needs. But we often choose foods based on their basic function: calories in. What if I told you that food had a secret language? That it can guide us to choose what will nourish and heal our bodies and minds? That language is flavor.

Flavor is about so much more than "does this taste good?" Flavor teaches us all about the actions of foods. The most recognizable flavors are sweet, sour, bitter, pungent and salty. Like people, foods are complex; one single food item may offer more than one of these flavor profiles. Flavors can prompt specific physiological responses, such as salivation and the release of gastric juices to promote digestion. Some flavors may suggest specific characteristics; for example, sour can be indicative of antioxidant action. Other flavors are so subtle that you might not even perceive any flavor—but that blandness has medicinal virtue.

This concept of flavor energetics focuses on how foods and herbs heal. You use your senses, particularly those of smell and taste, and you rely on your own intuition—how foods make you feel.

Truth be told, our bodies already know how to do this. But we need to listen to our bodies and use our senses—instead of reaching for pharmaceuticals—to heal what ails us. If this book teaches you nothing else, I hope that it teaches you that you alone know best what your body needs.

Sour

What comes to mind when you think of sour foods? Lemons, oranges, Granny Smith apples, vinegar? Sour foods are the foods that make you pucker. Sour flavors are tart and induce salivation. Energetically speaking, sour flavors make me think of flow, fluid and movement.

Sour foods are often loaded with the antioxidants and vitamins that are essential to protecting cells. They play a vital role in maintaining a strong immune system, both helping to prevent acute illness and shorten the duration of symptoms. Sour food can also encourage detoxification and encourage digestion, while also protecting skin from damaging free radicals.

Sour Flavor Food Profile

Fruits

- Berries
- Cherries
- Grapefruit
- Grapes
- Green apple
- Kiwi
- Kumquats
- Lemons
- Limes
- Nectarines
- Oranges
- Peaches
- Pineapple
- Plums
- Starfruit
- Tamarind
- Tomato

Vegetables

- Fermented and pickled vegetables

Dairy

- Buttermilk
- Cultured butter
- Kefir
- Some fresh cultured cheeses
- Sour cream
- Yogurt

Grains

- Sourdough and traditionally fermented breads

Herbs & Spices

- Five-flavor berry (schisandra)
- Hawthorn berry
- Rose hip
- Wood sorrel

Other

- Fermentation brine
- Fermented sodas
- Kombucha
- Vinegar

Pungent

Think spicy. Think heat. These foods make your eyes open wide. They make your tongue dance from pleasure—and maybe a little pain. Pungent herbs and spices include garlic, chile peppers, horseradish and black pepper. Less obvious pungent foods are cinnamon, ginger, allspice and clove.

Pungent foods are barrier breakers. These are the diffusive herbs, spices and foods that break up stagnancy and get things moving. Reach for pungent foods when you have an upset stomach, stuffed-up sinuses or pelvic fullness and cramping. Pungent foods can increase digestion—and can even act as an aphrodisiac!

Pungent Flavor Food Profile

Fruits
- Quince (ripe)

Vegetables
- Arugula
- Chile peppers
- Garlic
- Leeks
- Onions
- Radishes
- Scallions

Grains
- Buckwheat
- Spelt

Herbs & Spices
- Allspice
- Anise
- Bee balm
- Black pepper
- Cayenne
- Cinnamon
- Cloves
- Ginger
- Horseradish
- Mustard
- Nutmeg
- Oregano
- Paprika
- Red pepper flakes
- Thyme
- Turmeric

Bitter

Oh, bitter . . . you have an undeserved bad reputation. And your general absence from the modern diet is a serious problem. Dark chocolate and coffee remain fan favorites, but dark leafy greens, radicchio, endive and eggplant—not so much. Bitter foods may take a little cajoling to make them culinary masterpieces, but they are extremely important to the daily diet.

Bitter foods are perfect for digestion—and it is vital that we taste the bitterness. When we eat something bitter, a cascade of physiological responses takes place. This triggers the release of gastric juice and bile, essential for the digestion of rich foods and heavy fats. A lightly dressed salad of bitter greens may be just the ticket to protecting yourself from indigestion. Additionally, bitter foods, such as tea, tone and tighten mucus membranes, making them appropriate for treating coughs and diarrhea.

Bitter Flavor Food Profile

Fruits
- Citrus zest and pith
- Grapes
- Persimmon (unripe)

Vegetables
- Artichokes
- Beet tops
- Bitter melon
- Chicory
- Collards
- Cucumber
- Eggplant
- Endive
- Kale
- Radicchio

Grains & Seeds
- Amaranth
- Millet
- Quinoa

Herbs & Spices
- Bay
- Chervil
- Dandelion
- Hops
- Mugwort
- Rosemary
- Saffron
- Sage
- Turmeric
- Wild lettuce
- Wormwood

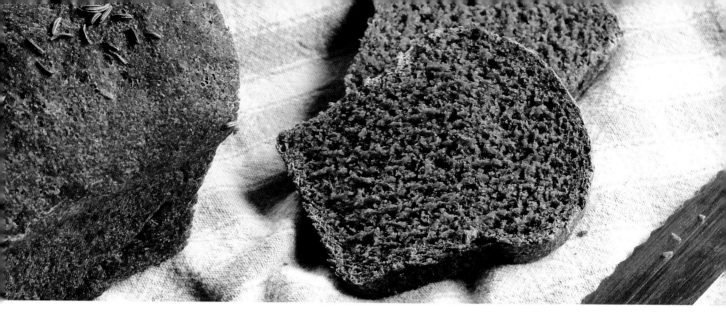

Sweet

When herbalists talk about sweet as a flavor, we aren't just referring to the sugary, candy-like flavor that you may be thinking of. We mean sweet in a broader sense. In fact, sweet can be rather bland and one dimensional. It can even be boring if not prepared with insight and creativity.

Sweet foods are typically carbohydrate-rich, sometimes mucilaginous and even a bit starchy. Oats and various other grains might be considered sweet, as are some vegetables such as corn, beets, potatoes and okra. Fruit is also sweet. Even milk and cream possess the nourishment that the sweet flavor profile suggests.

Sweet foods are typically nutrient-dense foods, although modern milling and breeding may have diluted the nutrient value of these foods. Seek out heirloom grains for complex nutrition. Try mushrooms for immunity-modulating polysaccharides.

Sweet Flavor Food Profile

Fruits

- Apples
- Bananas
- Dates
- Figs
- Paw paws
- Pears

Vegetables

- Beans
- Beets
- Carrots
- Corn
- Lentils
- Okra
- Potatoes
- Pumpkin and winter squash
- Sweet potatoes and yams
- Zucchini and summer squash

Dairy

- Cream
- Milk
- Sweet cream butter

Grains & Seeds

- Cashews
- Flax
- Oats
- Pumpkin seeds
- Rice
- Sesame seeds
- Sunflower seeds
- Wheat

Meats & Eggs

- Chicken (white meat)
- Pork

Herbs & Spices

- Allspice
- Basil
- Cinnamon
- Fennel
- Fenugreek
- Mint

Other

- Stevia
- Vanilla

Salty

Salty is a flavor profile that may not be what you think it is. Salty foods often taste mineral-like, even slightly metallic. Even a sweet banana has metallic notes indicative of its high potassium content! Salty foods also may have a varying degree of salinity, from seaweed to spinach to stinging nettle. The category also includes meat and seafood—both containing a variety of important vitamins and minerals that are rare in the plant world.

Salty foods are important in the restoration of electrolytes. After illness or strenuous exercise, your body needs these foods to bring back the balance of minerals such as sodium, potassium and magnesium. Salty foods also can help regulate the body's natural water content—retaining fluid and minerals where they are needed and sending any excess to be excreted.

Salty Flavor Food Profile

Fruits

- Banana
- Cantaloupe
- Coconut
- Honeydew melon
- Watermelon

Vegetables

- Brined and fermented vegetables
- Celery
- Green beans

- Seaweed
- Spinach

Dairy

- Aged cheeses

Meats & Eggs

- Dark-fleshed poultry and fowl
- Eggs
- Organ meat
- Red meat & game
- Seafood

Herbs & Spices

- Alfalfa
- Clover
- Nettle
- Raspberry leaf
- Salt, including sea salt, kosher salt, Himalayan salt and artisanal salt

Other

- Soy sauce
- Tamari

The key to a healthy diet is a balance of all of these flavors. By learning about them, you can make informed food choices to address your acute and chronic concerns.

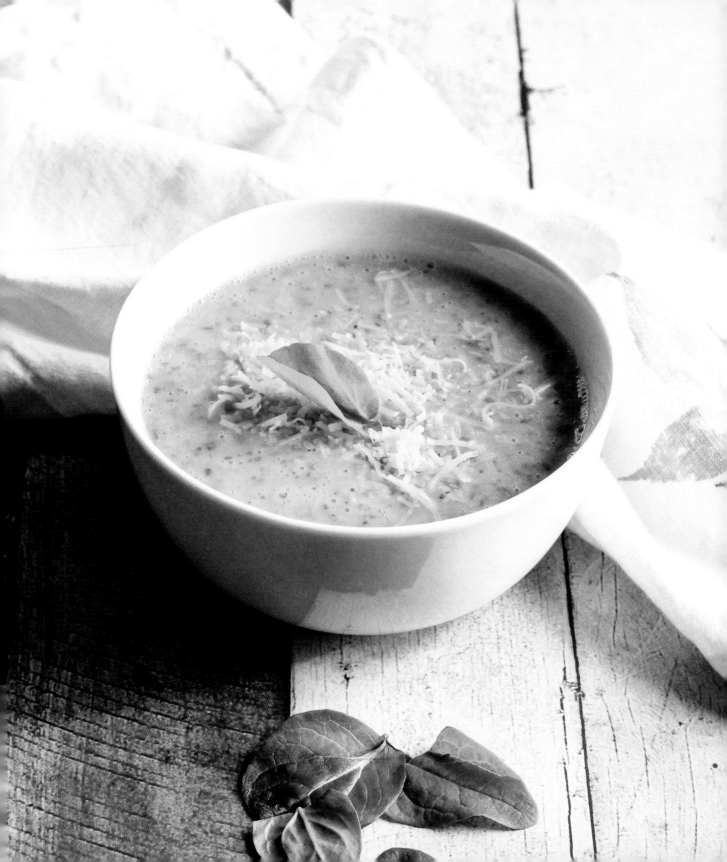

ONE

RECIPES TO

RECHARGE & RESET

Detoxification is a trendy word that entices people into impulse purchases and quick-fix solutions. The truth is that our bodies are detoxifying every single day, and we are purging contaminants and toxic substances constantly. Our bodies rely on the organs of elimination—the liver, skin, lungs, digestive system and urinary system—to maintain good health.

For a variety of reasons, such as poor food choices, environmental factors, surgery, medications and hormonal imbalances, these organs of elimination may become sluggish. When they are slow to respond, we tend to feel cloudy, dumpy and altogether unwell.

There is a whole host of revitalizing herbs and foods to encourage the natural detoxification process. Look for sour, pungent and bitter foods. These are the movers and the shakers in the flavor world.

Add pungent garlic and ginger, bitter turmeric and even the slightly sour cilantro to your meal plan to reboot your body. Encourage a clear complexion with a creamy Roasted Cauliflower Soup (page 25). Quench your thirst with a cold glass of Honey-Fermented Turmeric Ginger Ale (page 30) to show your liver some extra TLC. Or have a serving of Cilantro-Lime Rice (page 21) to help purge heavy metals from your body.

These recipes support your body's natural detoxification functions, and they help you press restart on your health.

Parsley is far more than a garnish placed thoughtlessly on a plate, folks. This lovely sprig of green is one of the most useful herbs in the kitchen. Its benefits include reducing inflammation and supporting the immune system. Parsley is also nutrient-rich, and it assists the body's natural detoxification process.

Chimichurri is a popular Argentinian sauce or marinade traditionally made with oil. This spicy chimichurri compound butter is perfect served over a grilled flank steak, and it's equally at home slathered into a fluffy baked potato. Garlic, red pepper flakes and parsley make a bright, flavorful compound butter that will titillate your taste buds and contribute to good health.

FLANK STEAK WITH CHIMICHURRI COMPOUND BUTTER

Flavor Profile: *Pungent, Bitter, Salty*

Serves: *4 to 6*

½ cup (112 g) butter, softened to room temperature

4–6 cloves garlic, finely minced

1 cup (60 g) firmly packed fresh flat-leaf parsley, trimmed of thick stems and minced

2 tbsp (10 g) fresh oregano leaves, minced (or 2 tsp [2 g] dried oregano)

¼–½ tsp red pepper flakes

Salt & freshly ground pepper, to taste

1½–2 lb (680–900 g) flank or flat iron steak

In a medium-sized bowl, combine the softened butter with the garlic, parsley, oregano and red pepper flakes. Stir well and taste for seasoning, adding salt and pepper to taste. Scoop the compound butter onto plastic film or waxed paper. Using the film or paper, form a log with the butter, wrap and refrigerate for at least 30 minutes or until firm. You want a well-chilled compound butter so that it melts slowly across the finished meat.

To prepare the steak, heat up the grill to medium-high. Pound the steak with a tenderizing mallet on both sides. Pat it dry with a paper towel and season with salt and pepper on both sides. Grill over medium-high heat for 5 to 7 minutes on each side for medium rare. Alternately, cook under the broiler until desired doneness is reached. Remove it from the heat and allow the meat to rest for 7 to 10 minutes before slicing against the grain.

Slice the chimichurri compound butter into rounds. Place them over warm slices of the meat to melt.

The chimichurri butter can be frozen for up to 6 months.

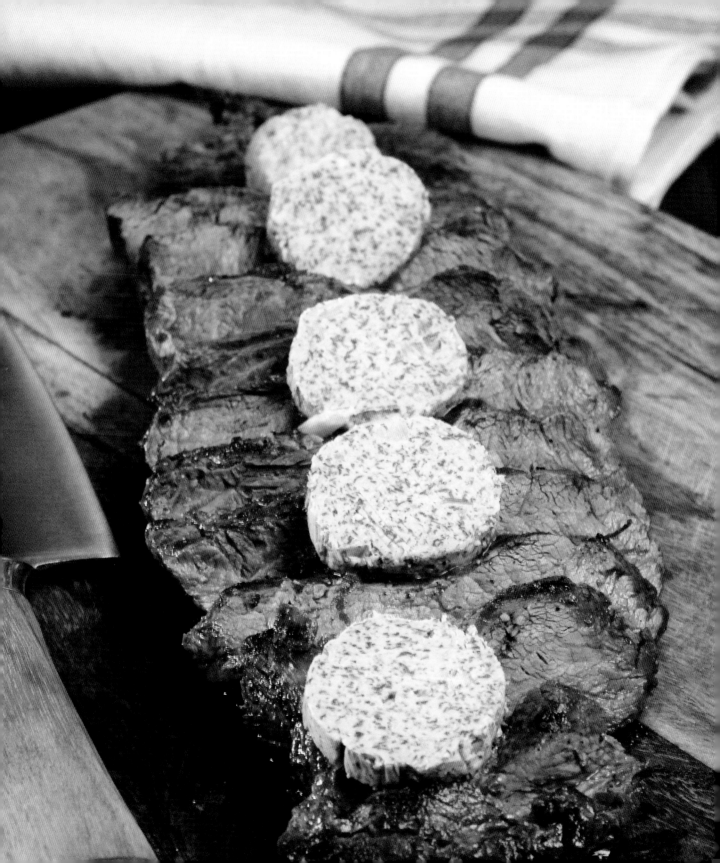

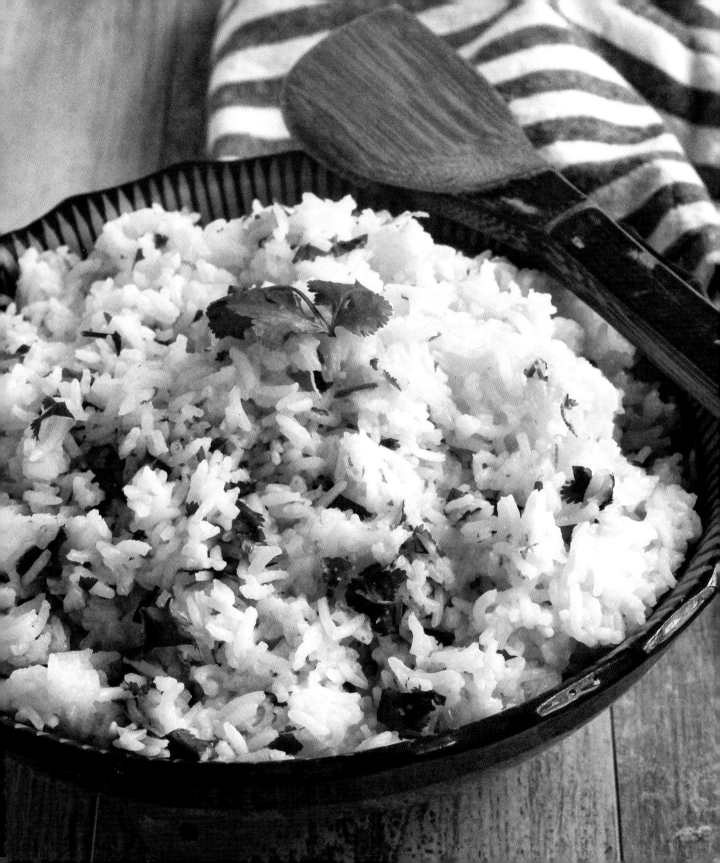

Yes, this is my version of the famous rice dish served at a popular fast-dining restaurant. But I turned the volume up—A LOT. This rice is full of cilantro and lots of lime.

Cilantro is a chief herb used in ridding the body of heavy metals, making it an excellent herb for detoxification. Some object to the flavor and call it "soapy"; others love cilantro and can't get enough of it. I definitely belong to the latter camp.

Did you know that cilantro stems are full of flavor? Chop them up and include them. I like to use lime juice and lime zest, saving the zest to add just before serving so that it retains its bright citrusy aromatics. Be sure to soak and rinse your rice thoroughly to produce a light, fluffy result. This rice perfectly complements the Pinto Beans with Cumin & Epazote (page 102).

CILANTRO-LIME RICE

Flavor Profile: *Pungent, Sweet*

Serves: *4 to 6*

1 cup (185 g) basmati or long-grain white rice

1½ cups (355 ml) water, plus more for soaking the rice

½ cup (120 ml) fresh lime juice

1 tsp salt

1½ cups (24 g) chopped cilantro

Zest of 1 lime

In a medium-sized bowl, soak the rice in enough cool water to cover for about 20 minutes. Drain it in a fine-mesh sieve. Rinse the rice well with cool water, until the water draining away is clear.

In a medium-sized saucepan, add the water, lime juice, salt and rinsed rice. Bring it to a low boil over medium-high heat. When boiling, reduce the heat to low and cover. Cook for about 20 minutes, until the rice is tender.

Fluff the rice with a fork and add the cilantro and lime zest. Fluff well to combine. Serve immediately.

Avocados are a true treat. These green treasures are so incredibly nutritious and oh-so-very tasty! They boast riboflavin, niacin, magnesium, potassium, folate, lutein, beta-carotene, omega-3 fatty acids, pantothenic acid, as well as vitamins C, E and K. Full of healthy fats, these creamy fruits support health and wellness while contributing to a feeling of fullness.

This soup is perfect for those needing a nourishing meal on a hot day. The addition of cilantro offers a detoxifying aspect: cilantro is indicated for the purging of toxic heavy metals from the body. Served for lunch or dinner, this hits all the nutrition marks for a well-rounded meal. It is also light on protein, gentle on the kidneys and perfect for those following Keto-style diets.

CHILLED AVOCADO SOUP

Flavor Profile: *Sweet, Pungent, Sour*
Serves: *4 to 6*

3 tbsp (45 ml) extra-virgin olive oil

1 cup (160 g) diced white onion

3 cloves garlic, minced

1 serrano chile, stemmed, seeded and diced

4 avocados, firm but yielding to gentle pressure

4 cups (940 ml) vegetable broth

2 cups (210 g) seeded, diced cucumber

¼ cup (60 ml) fresh lemon juice

¼ cup (4 g) chopped fresh cilantro leaves

½ cup (100 g) plain Greek yogurt

In a large skillet, heat the olive oil over medium-high heat. Add the onion, garlic and chile and sauté until softened and the onions are translucent, about 5 to 7 minutes. Set them aside and allow to cool.

In a blender, add the onion mixture along with the avocados, broth, cucumber, lemon juice, cilantro and yogurt. Blend on high until completely smooth and creamy, about 30 seconds to 1 minute. Chill the soup completely in the refrigerator for at least 2 hours. When ready to serve, ladle it into bowls.

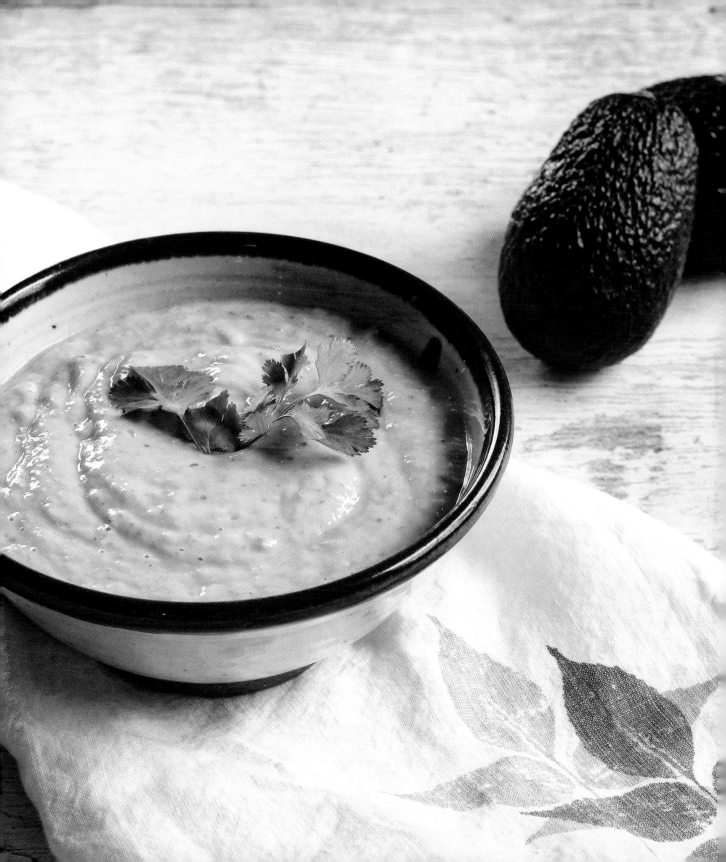

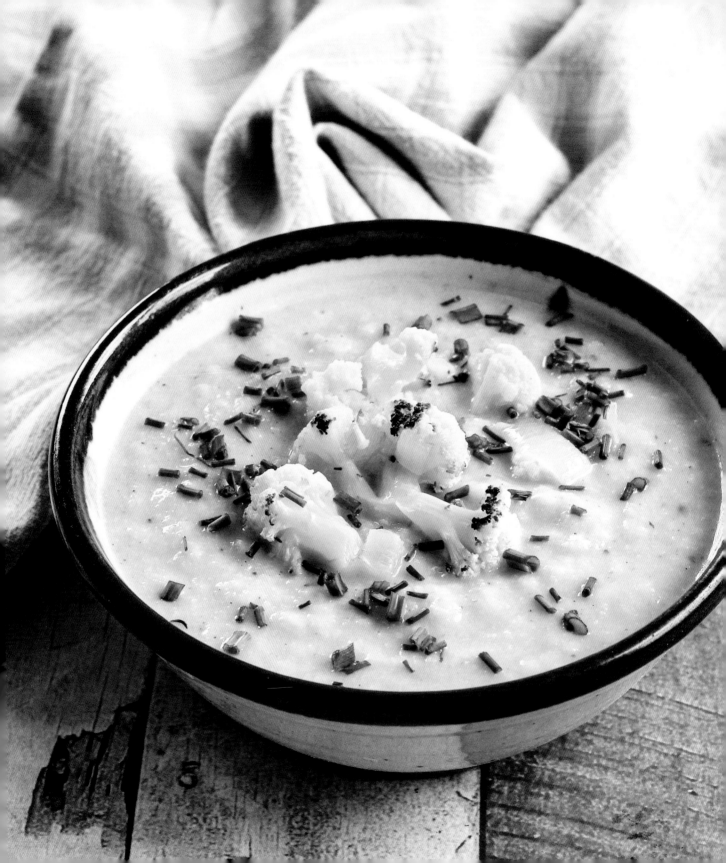

I was well into my twenties before I learned to appreciate cauliflower—and I am so glad that I did. This bland and oddly textured food is totally transformed when it is roasted, and it becomes a rich, buttery and nutty meal.

High in fiber, as well as B-complex and C vitamins, the humble cauliflower is antioxidant and anti-inflammatory—both qualities that contribute to general good health and a radiant complexion. Cauliflower is an abundant source of sulfur, which is thought to help reduce breakouts. Additionally, garlic and cauliflower are a pair of potent liver detoxifiers, speeding the body's natural elimination of stored toxins. Adding bone broth to this soup works to increase collagen-supporting benefits, while the whole dish favors a happy, detoxified liver. This meal is easy to make vegan, and it is a perfect meal for busy weeknights.

ROASTED CAULIFLOWER SOUP

Flavor Profile: *Bitter, Sweet, Salty*

Serves: *4*

1 large head cauliflower, cut into florets and stem, chopped

1 medium onion, chopped

4–5 cloves garlic, crushed

4 tbsp (60 ml) extra-virgin olive oil, divided

4 cups (940 ml) vegetable or Bone Broth with Bone-Building Herbs (page 148)

½ cup (120 ml) heavy cream (optional)

Salt & freshly ground pepper, to taste

¼ cup (12 g) freshly snipped chives, for garnish

Preheat your oven to 425°F (220°C, or gas mark 7). Toss the cauliflower, onion and garlic with 2 tablespoons (30 ml) of olive oil. Spread the vegetables evenly on a rimmed baking sheet. Roast for about 20 minutes, or until the cauliflower is golden brown. Remove them from the oven.

Place the roasted vegetables in a medium-sized saucepan, reserving ¼ cup (25 g) of the smallest floret bits and pieces for garnish. Add the broth and bring it to a simmer over medium heat. Reduce the heat to medium-low. Continue to simmer with the lid on for about 20 minutes, or until the cauliflower is quite tender. Remove the pan from the heat.

Blend the vegetables to a smooth puree in a blender or using an immersion blender. While the blender is running, add the remaining 2 tablespoons (30 ml) of olive oil to emulsify. Stir in the heavy cream, if using, and season with salt and pepper to taste.

Ladle into bowls and garnish with the chives and reserved floret pieces.

If it is good enough for Popeye, it's good enough for me. The nutritional aspect of spinach was indoctrinated into me from early childhood by way of cartoons. And, truth be told, I've always liked spinach anyway. Those emerald-green leaves are a powerhouse. Packed with vitamins A, C and K, along with calcium, iron, folate, quercetin and lutein—spinach really has it all.

Peppery watercress adds bite and depth of flavor, and it offers a nutrient profile that is similar to spinach. Together, spinach and watercress make for a delicious, nutritious soup for folks who are feeling depleted or who are recovering from injury, illness or surgery. This nourishing soup will replenish your body and mind.

SPINACH & WATERCRESS SOUP

Flavor Profile: *Bitter, Salty, Pungent*

Serves: *4 to 6*

2 leeks

2 tbsp (28 g) butter

2–3 cloves garlic, minced

4 cups (940 ml) chicken or vegetable stock

2 large russet potatoes, peeled and diced (½ inch [1.3 cm])

3 cups (90 g) packed spinach leaves

1 cup (30 g) packed watercress leaves

Juice and zest of 1 lemon

2 cups (475 ml) heavy cream

Salt & freshly ground pepper, to taste

Sour cream or crème fraîche, for garnish (optional)

Aged cheese such as Parmesan, for garnish (optional)

Trim the root and dark green ends from the leeks, then slice lengthwise. Slice them thinly and divide the rings. Soak the leeks in cool water to allow any sand and dirt to dislodge and sink while the leeks float on the surface of the water. To drain, gently lift the floating leeks from the water without disturbing the dirt below; set them aside.

In a large stockpot over medium heat, add the butter, drained leeks and garlic. Sauté until they're translucent, soft and fragrant, about 5 to 7 minutes. Add the stock and potatoes. Simmer for about 15 to 20 minutes, or until the potatoes are tender and are easily pierced with a fork.

Add the spinach, watercress, lemon juice and zest, and return them to a simmer. Continue to simmer for at least 5 to 10 minutes, until the greens are tender.

Remove the pot from the heat and add the heavy cream. Blend it to a smooth puree in batches in a blender or using an immersion blender.

Season with salt and pepper to taste. Ladle the soup into serving bowls and garnish with sour cream and cheese, if desired.

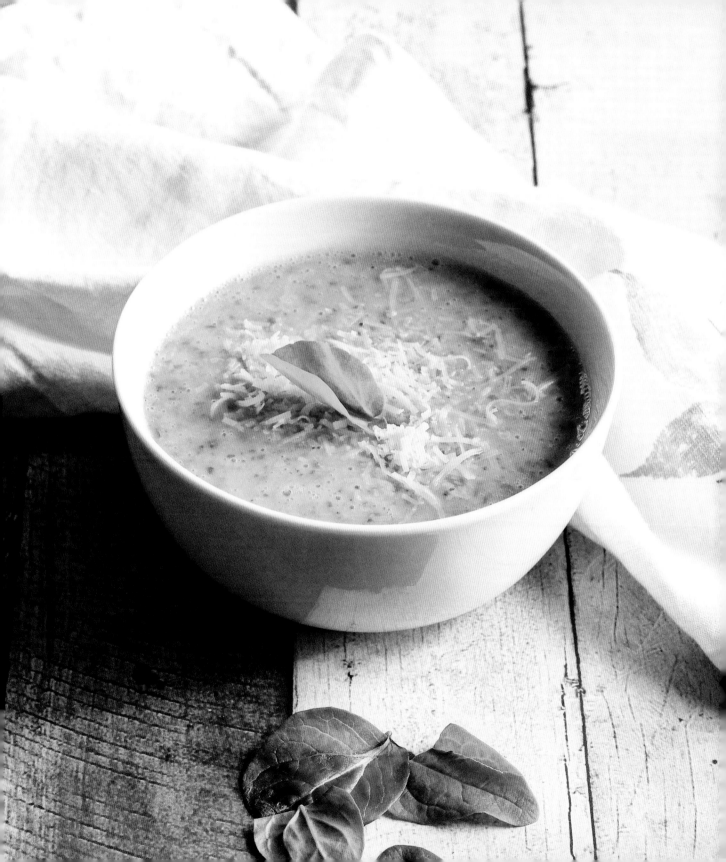

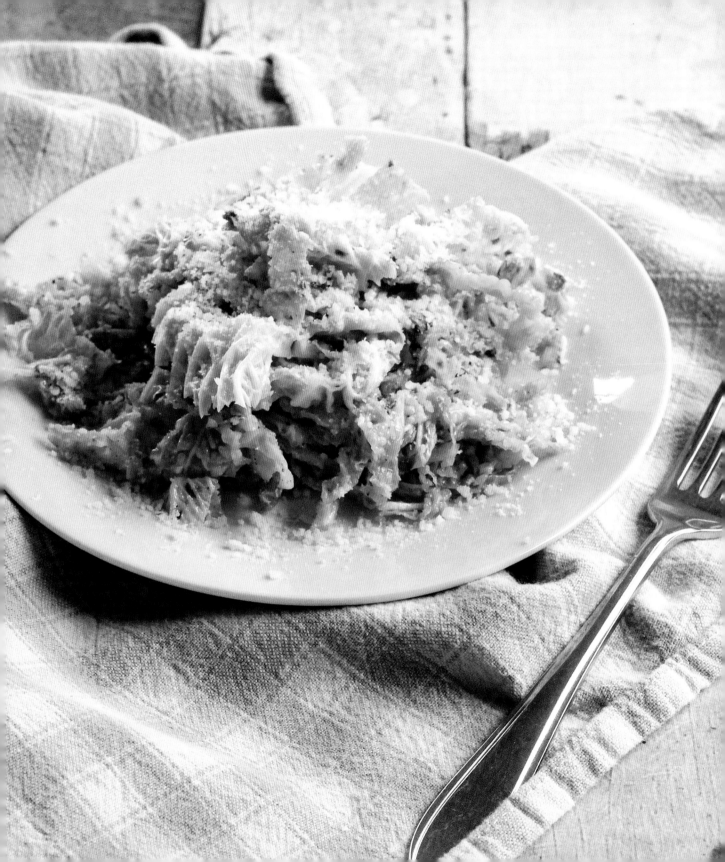

Cabbage is a grade-A detoxifier of the liver. It also promotes excellent digestion and boosts kidney function. Combined with garlic, these actions are amplified. Frequent meals with this combination are sure to result in a light, healthy feeling and a fresh, clear complexion.

Some folks may cringe a bit at the thought of anchovies, but I promise you that they will not create a strong fish flavor. Instead, a few fillets melt into the butter and add an umami-rich depth of flavor that somehow makes these "noodles" taste more like a meal! I prefer to use crinkly Savoy cabbage for this recipe as the leaves offer a tender and interesting texture.

CABBAGE "NOODLES" WITH GARLIC & ANCHOVIES

Flavor Profile: *Sour, Salty, Pungent*

Serves: *4 to 6*

5–6 cloves garlic, minced

¼ cup (60 ml) extra-virgin olive oil or butter

7–8 anchovy fillets

1 small Savoy cabbage, halved, cored and sliced thinly

Salt & freshly ground pepper, to taste

Large pinch of red pepper flakes, to taste

¼ cup (20 g) freshly grated Pecorino Romano cheese

In a large skillet over medium-low heat, cook the garlic in the olive oil, until just fragrant, about 1 to 2 minutes. Do not burn or brown the garlic; adjust the heat so that your garlic becomes fragrant but does not darken significantly.

In a small bowl or ramekin, mash the anchovy fillets with a fork. Add the anchovies to the garlic and cook for about 1 to 2 minutes.

Add the sliced cabbage by the handful, allowing each addition to wilt slightly before adding the next. Continue until all the cabbage has been added and becomes tender, 2 to 4 minutes.

Remove the skillet from the heat. Season with salt, pepper and red pepper flakes, to taste. Toss it well with the cheese.

Turmeric is often touted for its extraordinary anti-inflammatory actions, but any mention of turmeric should also extol its liver-loving virtues. Turmeric is one of the only substances that promotes both stages of the liver's natural detoxification process. When the liver is at its peak performance, the rest of the body often follows suit.

Despite turmeric's many health benefits, it is a recalcitrant character. It is often suggested to be taken with black pepper, which dramatically increases the bioavailability of its active constituents. Another way to coax out all the detoxifying benefits of turmeric is with fermentation. In this honey fermentation, we add ginger and black pepper for increased flavor and bioavailability.

Note: This ferment may contain trace amounts of alcohol.

HONEY-FERMENTED TURMERIC GINGER ALE

Flavor Profile: *Sour, Sweet, Pungent*

Makes: *1 cup (235 ml)*

1 cup (340 g) raw, unfiltered honey

¼ cup (25 g) fresh turmeric root, finely chopped

2 tbsp (12 g) fresh ginger root, finely chopped

1 tsp whole black peppercorns

16-oz (480-ml) swing top bottles

1–2 tbsp (20–40 g) honey per bottle

Unchlorinated, filtered water

Combine the honey, turmeric, ginger and peppercorns in a jar. Stir well to combine them. Cover it with a coffee filter or a square of cheesecloth secured with a rubber band. Stir it daily. Within a few days you should see signs of an active fermentation such as bubbles, foam and a notable thinning of the honey. Allow the mixture to ferment for 1 to 2 weeks, tasting to judge the flavor.

To make the turmeric and ginger ale, add 1 tablespoon (15 ml) of the fermented mixture, strained of its solids, to a swing top bottle. Add 1 to 2 tablespoons (20 to 40 g) of additional honey to the same bottle. Warm unchlorinated, filtered water to about 100°F (38°C) and fill the bottle to the shoulder. Cap and shake it well to combine.

Continue this secondary ferment at room temperature for 12 to 48 hours, depending on the temperature of the room. Check every 12 hours to assess carbonation levels and to prevent excessive pressure from building up in the bottles. When you like the carbonation levels, refrigerate the bottle and drink the ale within 7 to 10 days.

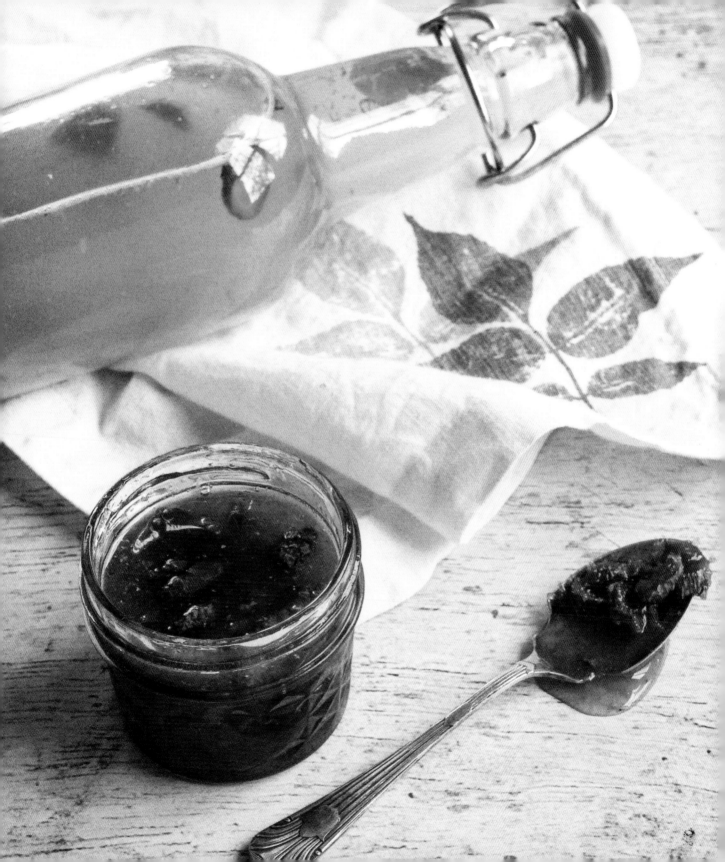

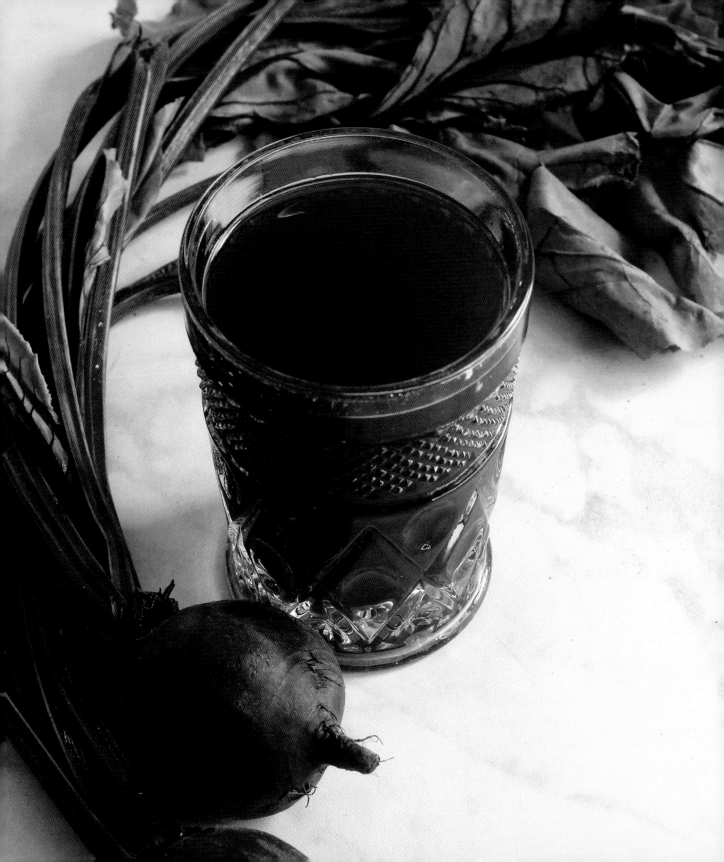

Let's just call this red Gatorade and make everybody give this healthy drink a try. Beets are full of powerful antioxidants, and beet kvass promotes good cardiovascular health and reduces oxidative stress on the liver. A 2018 review of a variety of plant-based treatments for alcoholic liver disease suggests that beets can play a significant role in improving and maintaining liver function.

This kvass is an excellent way to detoxify and restore the body with valuable electrolytes. Consumed daily, this beverage can earn a place in your wellness protocol. True, traditional beet kvass may be an acquired taste for some—too minerally and earthy for those not accustomed to this more Eastern European flavor profile. I bring in a bit of apple and aniseed to add some fresh, fruity and licorice-y flavor. The result is a pleasing and flavorful beverage that has a salinity similar to sports drinks.

BEET, APPLE & ANISEED KVASS

Flavor Profile: *Sour, Sweet, Pungent*

Makes: *About ½ gallon (1.9 L)*

2 tsp (10 g) unrefined sea salt

¼ cup (60 ml) whey drained from yogurt, or brine from a vegetable ferment such as Daikon Radish Kimchi (page 61) or sauerkraut

4 cups (940 ml) cool water

2 lb (900 g) beets, scrubbed clean

1 lb (450 g) apples, cored

1-gallon (3.8-L) jar

2 tbsp (12 g) aniseed

16-oz (480-ml) swing top bottles

Combine the salt and whey with the water. Set this aside.

Grate the beets and apples using a box grater. Pack them into a 1-gallon (3.8-L) jar and pour the whey starter culture over the apples and beets until they are covered by about 1 inch (2.5 cm) of liquid. Stir in the aniseed. Cover the jar with a lid outfitted with an airlock, or cover with several layers of cheesecloth or a coffee filter secured with a rubber band.

Ferment the kvass at room temperature for 5 to 7 days, tasting at day 4 or 5 for flavor. Strain, bottle and chill the liquid. The kvass will last 2 to 3 weeks in the refrigerator.

Herbalist Tips

To gather the whey used in this recipe, drain plain, unflavored yogurt in a fine-mesh sieve lined with muslin or cheesecloth, over a bowl. The whey collected in the bowl is an excellent source of lactic acid bacteria which promote fermentation. The thickened yogurt can be used as Greek yogurt or drained further for a cream cheese–like consistency. This process can take 4 to 12 hours, depending on the desired consistency.

While this is not a sweet ferment per se, the contents of your bottle may be under some pressure, so open with caution, especially if the kvass is warm or at room temperature.

I have been drinking green tea for most of my adult life, so when the matcha craze hit a few years back I was a bit bewildered. It's just green tea, right? Well, kind of. There is a whole ritual involved when it comes to preparing matcha tea. And these very acts of preparation are, in their own special way, an act of self-care.

By consuming green tea in the form of matcha, one is ingesting all the wonderful benefits of uncured *Camellia sinensis* leaves. Notably, matcha is loaded with powerful antioxidants and has a profound protective and detoxifying effect on the liver. These fun treats offer many of the benefits of matcha—in the form of a buttery cookie!

MATCHA & CASHEW SHORTBREAD

Flavor Profile: *Bitter, Sweet*

Makes: *About 2 dozen cookies*

½ cup plus 2 tbsp (140 g) unsalted butter, softened

¼ tsp almond extract

½ cup (100 g) sugar

1 cup (125 g) all-purpose flour

2 tbsp (12 g) matcha powder

⅛ tsp sea salt

⅓ cup (45 g) cashews, finely chopped

Preheat your oven to 325°F (170°C, or gas mark 3).

In the bowl of a stand mixer or with an electric beater, cream the butter, almond extract and sugar until fluffy. In a separate medium-sized bowl, sift together the all-purpose flour, matcha powder and salt. Stir the flour-matcha mixture into the butter mixture by hand, being careful not to overmix. Add the cashews and stir until the nuts are well distributed.

Scoop the dough onto plastic film or waxed paper, then form the dough into a 1½-inch (3.5-cm)-thick log. Wrap the log and freeze it for at least 30 minutes or up to 1 hour.

Remove the dough from the freezer. Cut the dough into slices about ¼ inch (6 mm) thick. Line two trays with parchment paper or silicone mats and arrange the slices about 2 inches (5 cm) apart. Bake for about 15 minutes, or until the edges of the cookies are very slightly golden.

Remove the trays from the oven and cool the shortbread completely on the baking sheets. Store the cookies in an airtight container for up to 1 week.

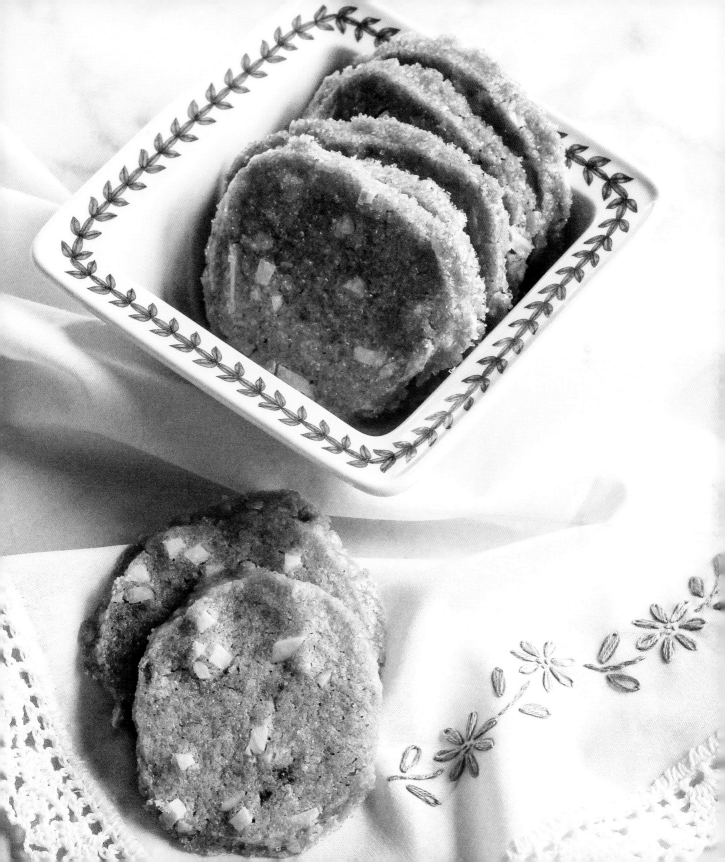

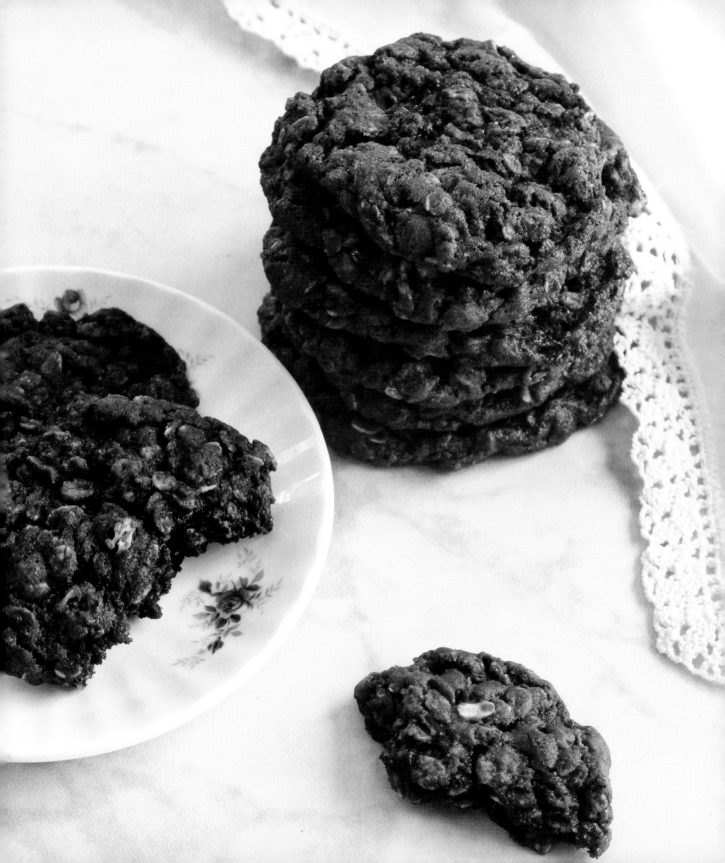

TWO

RECIPES FOR

RESTORATION & REPLENISHMENT

We all know the feeling: the depleted, crispy critter that we become in times of physical, mental and emotional stress. Self-care takes a backseat.

It doesn't have to be like this. And we often don't need expensive supplements to refill our empty tanks. In fact, nutrients are best absorbed as food. You hear that?— through what we eat. Vitamins, minerals and phytonutrients assimilate much more readily during the natural process of digestion.

Seek out salty and sweet flavor profiles when you need nourishment to help you rebalance and restore. These are the foods with vital nutrients, electrolytes and filling carbohydrates. You can find medicinal properties in common herbs and everyday spices, such as cinnamon, or experience the fortifying benefits of medicinal slippery elm. Try wild-sounding dulse flakes to season and thicken a dish—and provide a myriad of healing actions.

A Lemon Congee with Poached Eggs & Radish Microgreens (page 38) is a truly soul-filling meal on a cool day. Offer chewy Oatmeal, Molasses & Fenugreek Cookies (page 50) to a nursing mother. Or slip into the brine-y undersea world with a delicious Seaweed Salad (page 45).

Don't live life undernourished. Use this chapter to find the foods that will fill your body and restore your essence.

Refueling your body needn't be tedious or complex. In fact, simple recipes like this one come together quite easily—transforming yesterday's rice into a flavorful and filling breakfast.

The restorative benefits aren't just in the rice and the showy toppings. They are in the broth. I like to use a basic Bone Broth with Bone-Building Herbs (page 148), or a good homemade vegetable or mushroom broth. It should be fairly salty because the salinity of the broth helps our internal tissue to retain water and restore electrolyte balance.

The lemon and the spicy radish greens add brightness and complexity to the congee, while the runny yolk of a beautifully poached egg adds a special richness that can't be beat. This congee is a great breakfast, but can be enjoyed any time when you are feeling low on energy.

LEMON CONGEE WITH POACHED EGGS & RADISH MICROGREENS

Flavor Profile: *Salty, Sweet, Sour, Pungent*

Serves: *2*

1¾ cups (410 ml) Bone Broth with Bone-Building Herbs (page 148) or vegetable/mushroom stock

¼ cup (60 ml) fresh lemon juice

1 clove garlic, minced

1½ cups (235 g) cooked long-grain white rice (about ¾ cup [140 g] uncooked)

Zest of 1 lemon

Soy sauce, tamari or Himalayan sea salt

2 eggs

Distilled white vinegar

½ cup (17 g) loosely packed radish microgreens, for garnish

Add the broth, lemon juice and minced garlic to a medium-sized saucepan. Bring it to a boil over high heat. Reduce the heat to low and add the cooked rice. Cook uncovered for 15 to 20 minutes, stirring occasionally, until the rice starts to break apart and the broth has thickened. You may find that you need to add a small amount of liquid to prevent the mixture from becoming too thick; congee should have a stir-able, porridge-like texture. When the rice is tender, remove the congee from the heat. Stir in the lemon zest and season with soy sauce.

To poach your eggs, bring a small saucepan filled with water and a splash of distilled white vinegar to a steady simmer. Crack an egg into a small bowl or ramekin. Start stirring the water in a circular pattern to create a slight vortex in the middle of your pot. Quickly pour your egg into the center of the vortex; this will help the whites to wrap around the egg yolk. Cook the egg at a simmer for 1½ to 2 minutes, depending on how runny you want your egg yolk. After cooking, lift your egg with a slotted spoon and drain it on a paper towel. Repeat with the second egg.

Ladle the congee into serving bowls. Top each with an egg, cutting it in half to allow the yolk to spill out. Garnish with a generous amount of radish greens.

Herbalist Tip
This recipe calls for cooked rice. If you don't have any on hand, cook ¾ cup (140 g) of any long-grain, basmati or jasmine rice according to the package directions to produce about 1½ cups (235 g) of cooked rice.

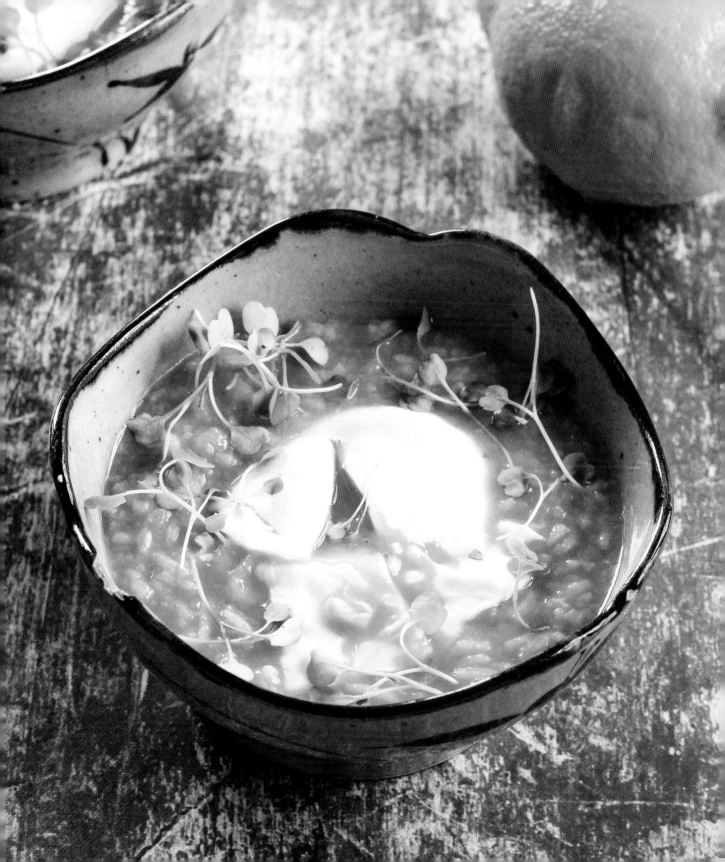

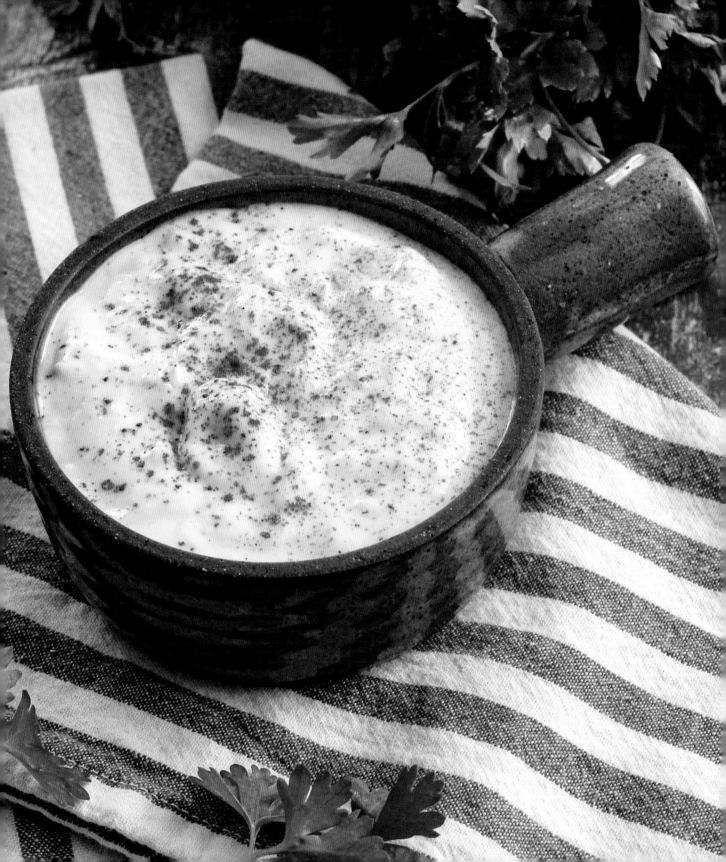

Nothing sticks to the ribs better on a cold winter day than a hearty bowl of clam chowder. This creamy soup has an abundance of potatoes, and the carrageenan-rich dulse flakes contribute a brine-y flavor.

Clams are an excellent choice for those looking for an iron-rich meal. A 3½-ounce (100-g) serving of clams contains 28 milligrams of iron; that's 155 percent of the recommended dietary allowance! Beef livers contain only a little over 6 milligrams. Clams are also far less susceptible to the contamination that is sometimes observed in other bivalves, such as mussels and oysters. Salty dulse, sometimes used to increase iodine levels and improve a sluggish thyroid, has an ample supply of vitamin B12, which is a difficult nutrient to find outside of animal products. Vitamin B12 is thought to improve energy, eyesight and red blood cell formation.

I developed this recipe keeping in mind the gluten and dairy sensitivities in my family. Brimming with minerals and thick with potatoes, this soup is lick-the-bowl good—and it's good for you.

GLUTEN-FREE CLAM CHOWDER

Flavor Profile: *Salty, Sweet*
Serves: *4 to 6*

4 slices bacon, minced

1 large onion, diced

4 ribs celery, diced

6 cups (900 g) peeled and diced russet potatoes

8 cups (1.9 L) water

1 lb (450 g) chopped clam meat

1 tsp Old Bay seasoning or other seasoned salt

2 tbsp (6 g) dulse flakes

1 cup (235 ml) half-and-half (optional)

Salt & freshly ground pepper, to taste

1 tbsp (3 g) snipped chives, for garnish (optional)

In a large stockpot, render the minced bacon over medium heat, about 7 to 10 minutes. When the bacon is browned and starting to crisp, remove it from the pan and drain it on a couple layers of paper towels.

Add the onion and celery to the bacon grease in the pan. Cook, stirring frequently, until they're translucent, about 5 to 7 minutes. Add the potatoes and water to the pot and turn up the heat to high. Boil the potatoes until tender, about 15 to 20 minutes. Turn off the heat and remove about half the potatoes using a slotted spoon. Using an immersion blender, puree the mixture until it's creamy.

Return the cooked potatoes to the pureed mixture and add the clam meat, Old Bay seasoning and dulse flakes. Turn the heat to medium-low and simmer, stirring occasionally, for 20 minutes. Stir in the half-and-half, if using. Season with salt and pepper to taste.

Ladle the chowder into bowls and garnish with a few pinches of chives, if desired.

How much more superfood can you get than quinoa and kale? This is like the hipster version of Caesar salad—and so much healthier. This is the perfect recipe for restoring the body. Kale offers an abundance of vitamins, minerals and phytonutrients, and quinoa acts as a perfect protein.

Dandelion leaves are a mineral-rich green with valuable nutrients, and they also aid in digestion. The sesame dressing lends nuttiness, and sesame oil and seeds are often used medicinally to help control inflammation and normalize hormones. Thinly sliced radishes offer this salad color and a peppery bite.

This salad gets better after sitting for a while, so make this a night ahead for a midday meal. Filling and nutrient-rich, it will keep your energy soaring for the rest of the day!

KALE & DANDELION SALAD WITH QUINOA

Flavor Profile: *Bitter, Salty, Pungent, Sour*

Serves: *2, generously*

2 cups (135 g) chopped kale, packed (I like tender-leaf cultivars such as Red Russian; remove the inner rib of sturdier cultivars.)

½ cup (28 g) fresh dandelion leaves (arugula is a good substitution if dandelion is out of season)

1 cup (116 g) thinly sliced radishes

1½ cups (278 g) cooked quinoa, cooled (see Herbalist Tip)

1 small clove garlic, minced

⅓ cup (80 ml) rice wine vinegar

3 tbsp (45 ml) soy sauce

½ cup (120 ml) toasted sesame seed oil

2 tbsp (16 g) toasted sesame seeds, for garnish

Sea salt, to taste

In a medium-sized bowl, mix the kale, dandelion leaves, radishes and quinoa until they're evenly distributed.

In a separate bowl, add the garlic, rice wine vinegar and soy sauce. Slowly whisk in the sesame oil to emulsify. You may need to whisk it again before adding it to the quinoa mixture.

Toss the kale-quinoa mixture with the dressing. Serve it garnished with toasted sesame seeds and season with sea salt to taste.

Herbalist Tip
Use precooked quinoa prepared according to package directions. Or rinse ¾ cup (128 g) of uncooked quinoa and bring 1½ cups (355 ml) of water to a simmer. Reduce the heat, cover and cook on low for about 20 minutes.

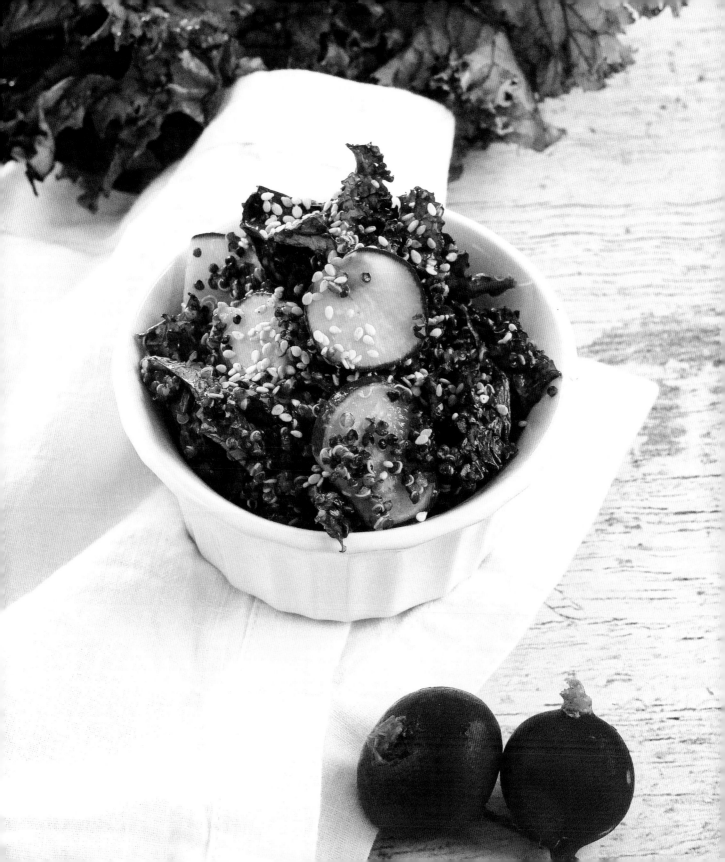

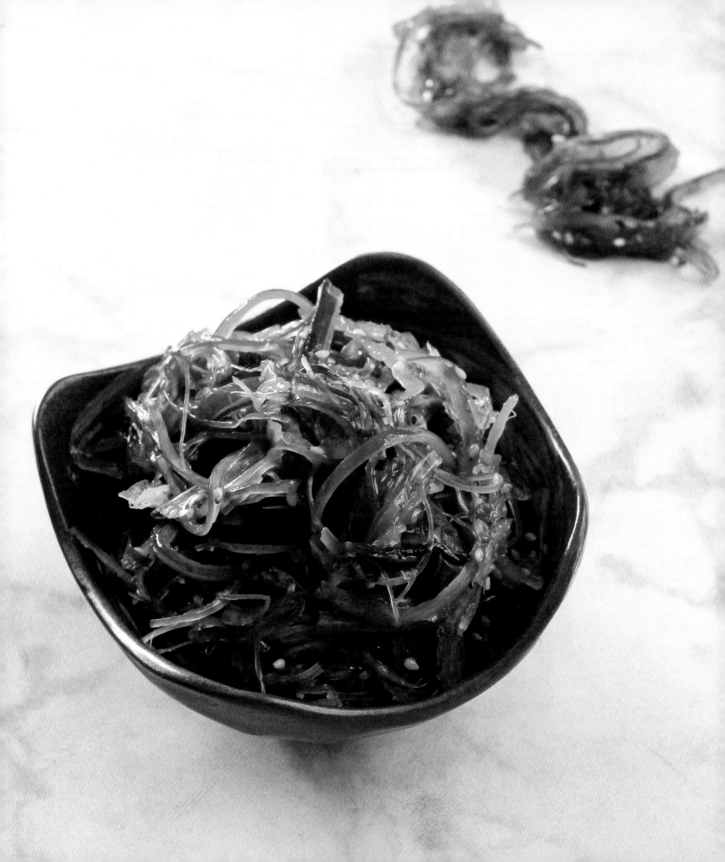

I crave the briny flavors of the ocean. My father's paternal line harks back only two generations to seafaring Scottish folk from the Outer Hebrides islands known for their rocky, meager landscape. I can only surmise that my not-so-distant ancestors scratched out subsistence using anything that the ocean would offer. Namely, seaweed.

While this recipe bears a far more Asian flavor profile, the underlying idea is the same—a salty dish, rich in minerals and complex phytonutrients. When we discuss the organs of elimination, we often seek herbs that assist with output. However, some of us need to balance our kidneys and urinary tract in the other direction. We need to retain. And dishes that boast a profound salinity help us to do just that.

This seaweed salad encourages our tissues to retain fluids and maintain a proper electrolyte balance. Simply eating a small bowl of this oceanic salad recharges the body, encourages water consumption and restores vitality. This dish serves as a light appetizer or as an accompaniment to Asian-inspired meals or sushi.

SEAWEED SALAD

Flavor Profile: *Salty, Pungent*

Serves: *4 to 6*

2½ cups (2 oz [56 g]) dried green wakame seaweed

2 tbsp (30 ml) rice wine vinegar

1 tsp sugar or honey

2 tsp (4 g) grated fresh ginger root

½ tsp wasabi powder or red pepper flakes

2 tsp (10 ml) soy sauce

1 tbsp (15 ml) roasted sesame oil

Sea salt, to taste (optional)

1 tbsp (8 g) sesame seeds, toasted, for garnish

Rehydrate the wakame seaweed by placing it in a bowl and covering it with an ample amount of cool water. When the wakame is rehydrated and tender, about 15 minutes, or according to package directions, drain it and pat it dry. Slice the seaweed thinly so that it resembles a tattered chiffonade.

In a separate bowl, whisk together the rice wine vinegar, sugar, ginger, wasabi powder and soy sauce. Slowly drizzle in the sesame oil while whisking vigorously to emulsify it.

Toss the wakame with the dressing. Taste it for seasoning, adjusting with sea salt if desired. Garnish it with toasted sesame seeds.

Hard work on the ole homestead during the heat of summer can leave me feeling completely drained, dried out and weak. What better way to replenish your fluids and electrolytes than with fruits and vegetables right out of the garden? Watermelon is high in potassium, a mineral ideal for infusing exhausted muscles with vitality once again. Adding basil oil as a garnish lends a variety of vitamins and minerals, as well as a calming influence after a hard day of work in the sun.

This watermelon gazpacho is simple to make. Just a rough chop and a quick blend, and this chilled soup is ready to serve. I love to serve this gazpacho as a light meal at lunch or as an appetizer for a larger meal, party or potluck.

HYDRATING WATERMELON GAZPACHO

Flavor Profile: *Salty, Sweet, Pungent*

Serves: *4*

1½ lb (680 g) seedless watermelon, cubed

1 lb (450 g) garden fresh tomatoes, roughly chopped

1 large bell pepper or 2–3 medium peppers, chopped

1 small onion, chopped

1 cucumber, peeled, seeded and chopped

2 cloves garlic, minced

2 slices bread, torn into shreds, OR 2 tbsp (22 g) chia seeds for gluten-free option

¾ cup (175 ml) extra-virgin olive oil, divided

Salt & freshly ground pepper, to taste

1 cup (24 g) fresh basil leaves

Combine the watermelon, tomatoes, pepper, onion, cucumber, garlic and bread in a large bowl, tossing well to combine them. Let the mixture sit in the bowl for 5 to10 minutes so that the bread can rehydrate. Blend to a smooth puree in a blender or using an immersion blender. When the gazpacho is smooth, slowly drizzle ¼ cup (60 ml) of the olive oil into the mixture while blending to emulsify it. Season with salt and pepper to taste. Chill the gazpacho for at least 1 hour.

To make the basil oil, blend the remaining ½ cup (120 ml) of olive oil and the basil in a blender for 1 to 2 minutes, until the basil is well incorporated into the oil. The oil should appear a deep emerald-green. Strain the oil through a few layers of cheesecloth.

Ladle the gazpacho into bowls and garnish it with swirls or dots of the basil oil. Serve immediately.

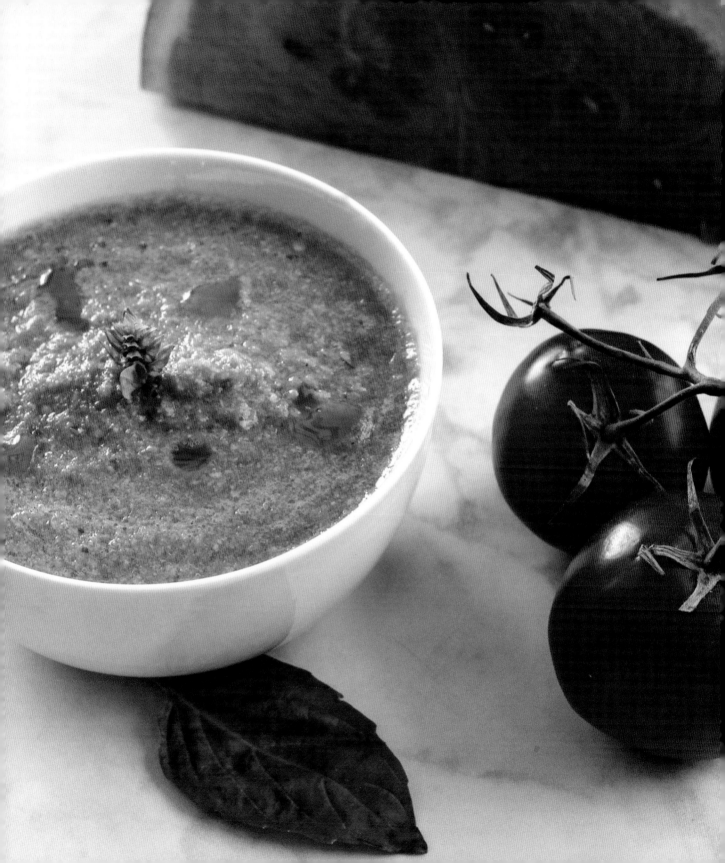

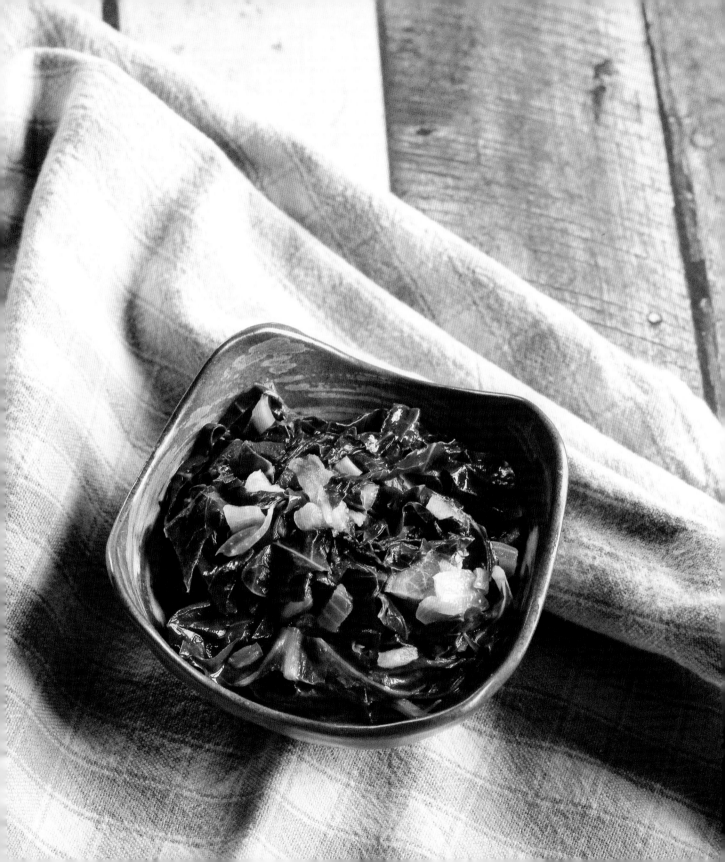

Humble food is the best food. The modest collard is one of the most nutritious members of the cruciferous family. Noted for its vitamin and mineral content, as well as an impressive array of phytonutrients, collards have a lot to offer. They have a staggering load of vitamins A, K and C, as well as minerals such as manganese and calcium. The slight bitterness and fiber content of the greens aid in the digestion of fats, and that cascade of benefits brought on by better digestion promotes healthy cholesterol levels.

These collards are first sautéed with garlic, a popular heart-friendly food, to add flavor. Then they're slowly braised in broth for a couple of hours until the greens are buttery and tender. I like to add a splash of unsweetened Fire Cider (page 65) before serving, to elevate and brighten the warm collards.

BRAISED COLLARD GREENS WITH GARLIC

Flavor Profile: *Bitter, Salty, Pungent*

Serves: *4 as a side dish*

4 slices thick-cut smoky bacon (optional)

1 tbsp (15 ml) reserved bacon fat or olive oil

2–3 cloves garlic, minced

4 cups (145 g) collard greens, cut in a chiffonade

1½ cups (355 ml) Bone Broth with Bone-Building Herbs (page 148; or use the broth of your choice)

1 tbsp (15 ml) vinegar or unsweetened Fire Cider (page 65)

Salt & freshly ground pepper, to taste

If using the bacon, dice it into small pieces. Brown the bacon over medium heat until crisp and well rendered, about 7 to 10 minutes. Remove the bacon pieces to a paper towel–lined plate to cool. Drain the bacon fat into a small container. You can omit this step if you are choosing the vegetarian/vegan options.

Heat the reserved bacon fat or olive oil over medium heat. Add the garlic and sauté for 1 to 2 minutes, until the garlic is fragrant. Add the collard greens and cook for another 3 to 4 minutes, until the collards start to go limp. Add the broth to the pan and cover it with a lid. Reduce the heat to low and simmer for about 2 hours.

After cooking, remove the lid and assess the moisture level. Your collards should have a fair bit of moisture and a "pan liquor," but they should not be soupy. If your greens are swimming in liquid, raise the heat and reduce to the desired moisture level. After the preferred liquid level is achieved, add the vinegar and season with salt and pepper to taste.

Postpartum care is vitally important to the health and well-being of new moms and their precious infants. This is a time of great nutritional need for both mama and baby to support and encourage lifelong good health. These cookies aren't just a sweet treat. I created this recipe with ingredients that replenish vital vitamins and minerals, as well as phytonutrients to encourage milk production. Blackstrap molasses is rich in calcium, iron and magnesium. It has a long-standing tradition of being used by new mothers to help increase breast milk production. Both oats and fenugreek are considered galactogogues—herbs that increase breastmilk production. They also contribute a moist and chewy texture and a bold maple-y flavor. Additionally, fenugreek helps to mitigate spikes in blood glucose levels and can help prevent the dreaded "sugar crash" after a sweet treat.

Make extra-large cookies so they can serve as a quick meal on the go for a nursing mama. A great gift idea would be a batch of this dough, individually portioned and frozen so that the cookies can be baked as needed!

OATMEAL, MOLASSES & FENUGREEK COOKIES FOR NURSING MAMAS

Flavor Profile: *Sweet, Pungent*
Makes: *About 2 dozen extra-large cookies*

2 cups (180 g) old-fashioned rolled oats

1 cup (125 g) all-purpose flour

1¼ tsp (5 g) baking soda

1 scant tsp salt

1 tsp cinnamon

1 tsp ground fenugreek

½ cup (112 g) butter, softened

1 cup (235 ml) maple syrup or sugar

½ cup (120 ml) blackstrap molasses

1 large egg

1 tsp vanilla extract

In a medium-sized bowl, mix together the rolled oats, flour, baking soda, salt, cinnamon and fenugreek. Set it aside.

In a stand mixer or using an electric beater, cream together the butter, maple syrup and molasses. Add the egg and vanilla and mix on high for about 40 seconds. Add the dry ingredients and beat until they're well combined. Chill for at least 30 minutes.

Preheat your oven to 375°F (190°C, or gas mark 5). Line a cookie sheet with parchment paper or a silicone mat. Using a large ice cream scoop, portion the chilled dough onto the cookie sheet, leaving 2 to 3 inches (5 to 7.5 cm) between the cookies. Bake for 9 to 12 minutes until golden. Remove them from the oven and cool on the cookie sheet for at least 4 minutes before removing and continuing to cool.

Store the cooled cookies in an airtight container for up to 1 week.

Herbalist Tip
Fenugreek is contraindicated for pregnancy; leave this out if making this recipe for a pregnant person.

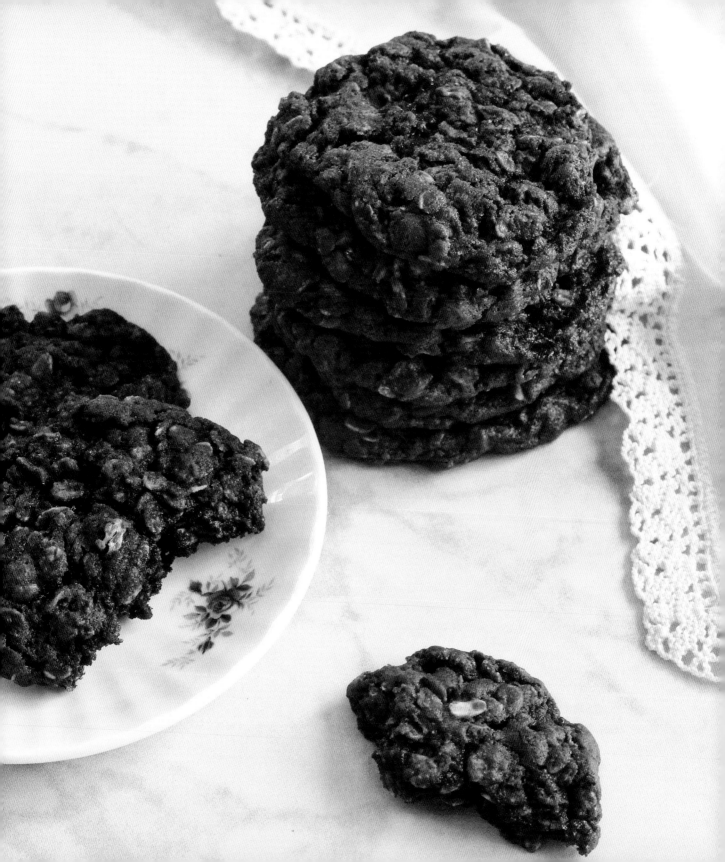

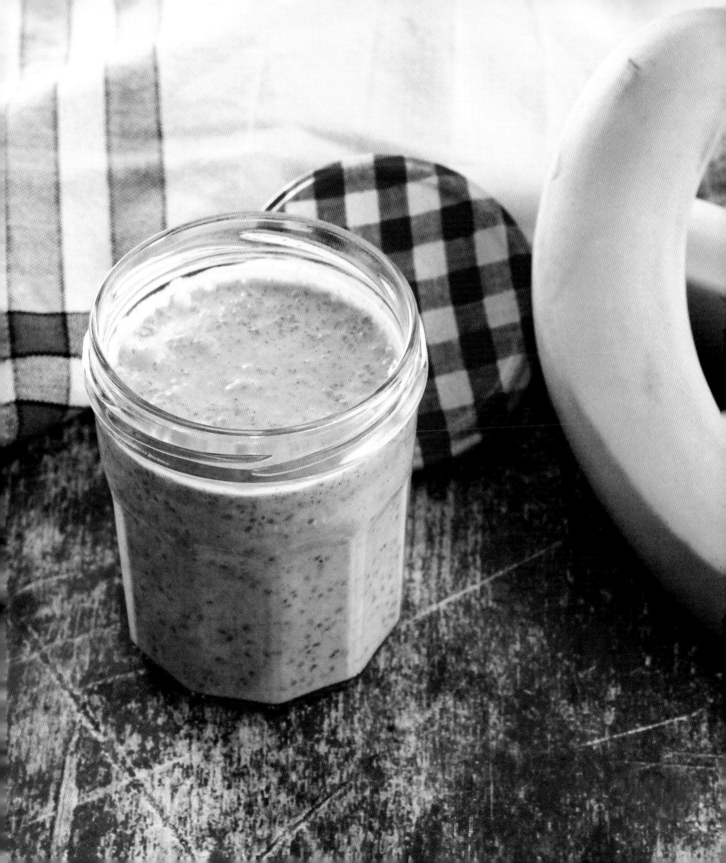

Chia seeds are a nutrient-dense superfood perfect for those looking to rest and recharge. Abundant in fiber, chia works its magic in the digestive system by promoting regular elimination and nourishing beneficial gut flora. Swelling to twelve times its weight upon hydration, chia seeds are also incredibly filling and they pack an enormous amount of nutrients within their tiny cell walls. Chia even contains an abundance of antioxidant omega-3 fatty acids, promoting good cardiovascular health and minimizing inflammation.

This breakfast pudding is a perfect morning meal for those looking for a plant-based way to start the day. Bananas offer sweetness and a boatload of potassium, while true cinnamon works alongside the chia to minimize spikes in blood sugar. This combination of chia and cinnamon sets the body up to sustain energy throughout the day and maintain healthy blood glucose levels. I personally find this pudding sufficiently sweet, but those who prefer more might opt for a small amount of maple syrup to sweeten things up.

CHIA, BANANA & CINNAMON BREAKFAST PUDDING

Flavor Profile: *Sweet, Salty*
Serves: *4 to 6*

2 cups (475 ml) full-fat unsweetened coconut milk

2 overripe bananas

1 tbsp (15 ml) maple syrup, or more to taste

½ tsp ground cinnamon

Pinch of salt

¼ cup (44 g) chia seeds

Sliced bananas and berries, for serving

In a blender, blend the coconut milk, bananas, maple syrup, cinnamon and salt until smooth.

In a medium-sized bowl, mix the chia seeds and the coconut-banana mixture. Allow the mixture to soak for 20 to 30 minutes. Stir well, spoon it into individual jars for serving and refrigerate for up to 48 hours. Serve with sliced bananas and fresh berries.

Oats are a nourishing grain that herbalists often use to help people who are recuperating from illness. Gentle on the stomach, a simple bowl of oatmeal is one of the first things I reach for after gastrointestinal distress. Soothing, nourishing and restorative, oats have it all.

This whole-grain granola turns the nutrition level up a few notches with the addition of flax, hemp hearts and seeds or nuts. Slippery elm root adds more digestive comfort to the granola and complements the flavor of my chosen sweetener—maple syrup. Slippery elm root is typically purchased ground; larger particles can be ground to a powder in a dedicated spice grinder or using a mortar and pestle.

Far from a bland cup of oatmeal, this nourishing granola is packed with flavor and texture, yet still offers the body that wholesome restorative quality that we have come to know and love. Try this granola over yogurt and fresh fruit. Dried fruit, such as cranberries and apricots, also make a tasty addition.

WHOLE-GRAIN GRANOLA WITH SLIPPERY ELM ROOT

Flavor Profile: *Sweet*

Makes: *A generous 6 cups (weight will vary)*

3 cups (270 g) old-fashioned rolled oats

½ cup (84 g) flaxseeds

½ cup (60 g) hemp hearts

½ cup (40 g) shredded, unsweetened coconut

1½ cups (weight will vary) raw nuts and/or seeds (such as walnuts, pumpkin seeds and/or sliced almonds)

2 tbsp (20 g) ground slippery elm root

1 tsp sea salt

1 tsp ground cinnamon

½ cup (120 ml) melted coconut oil or butter

½ cup (120 ml) maple syrup or honey

Preheat your oven to 325°F (170°C, or gas mark 3).

Toss the oats, flaxseeds, hemp hearts, coconut, nuts, slippery elm root, salt, cinnamon, coconut oil and maple syrup together in a large bowl until they're well combined.

Line a large sheet pan with parchment paper or a silicone mat. Spread the mixture out evenly. Press the mixture down firmly with a spatula to promote granola "clumps."

Bake for 25 to 30 minutes, until the granola is toasted and golden, stirring halfway through and pressing down firmly again. After baking, remove the granola from the oven and let it cool completely on the pan. When cool, break up large clumps with your hands. Store the granola in an airtight container for up to 2 weeks.

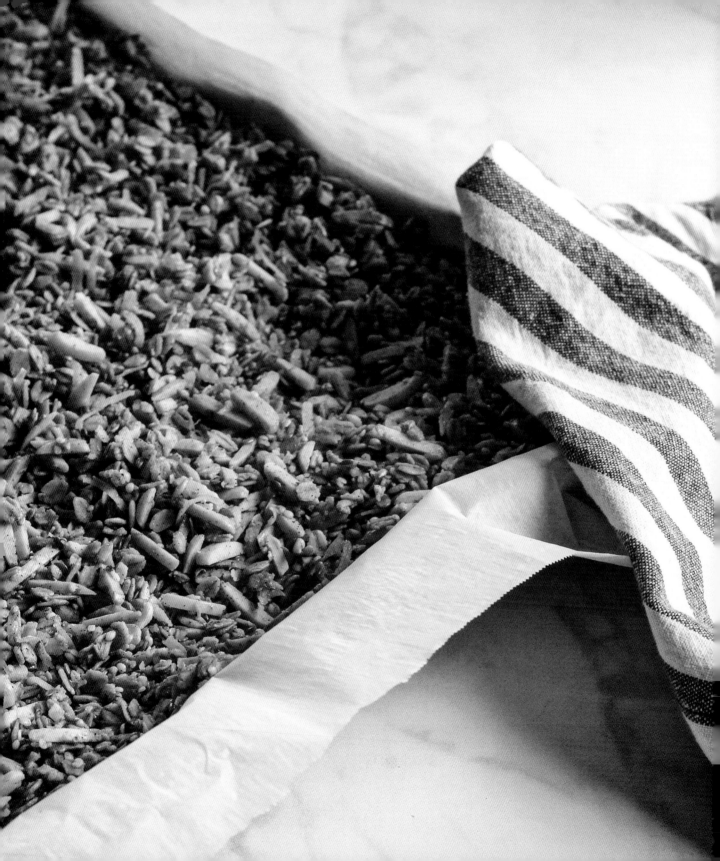

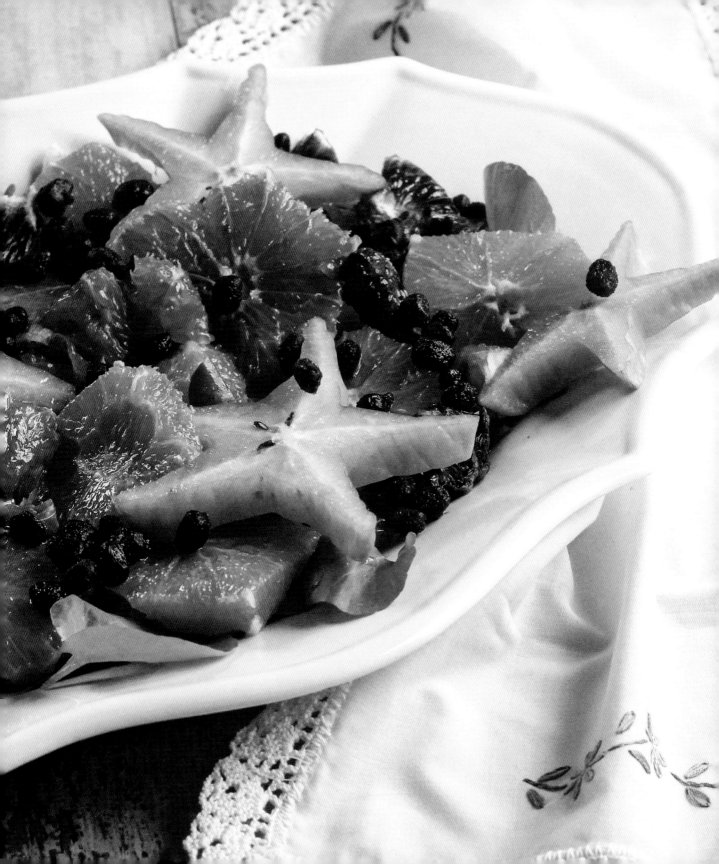

THREE

RECIPES FOR A
THRIVING IMMUNE SYSTEM

Immunity. It's a funny little thing. It is the invisible barrier that protects us. The immune system is a series of complex, and often poorly understood, organs. It is susceptible to damage, leaving us vulnerable to microbial attack. And beyond concerns about infection, some folks must contend with an immune system that goes haywire and starts harming instead of helping.

How do we care for this fragile and fickle bodily system? This is a system that needs protection and encouragement when under fire, and modulation when it is off-kilter. Excellent food choices are the key to maintaining good health and vitality.

Sour and pungent foods are right on target here, and garlic, ginger, lemongrass and citrus fruits take the spotlight. Take a swig of Fire Cider (page 65) when those around you start to sniffle. Break out the Thai Chicken Noodle Soup (page 58) when your glands are swollen and boggy. A bright Savory Citrus Salad (page 77) isn't just a feast for the eyes; it is an added layer of defense.

Sweet flavors—such as those found in medicinal and culinary mushrooms—play a supporting role in managing runaway immune systems. For those struggling with autoimmune disease, try the Cremini Mushrooms with Miso Butter (page 78) for immune-modulating polysaccharides.

Take charge of your immunity—and take a stand for your health!

Everybody loves a cup of chicken noodle soup when congestion, cough and that all-over body ache arrive. There is nothing wrong with basic chicken noodle soup, but I like to spice it up a bit when the first hint of sinus pressure hits.

Lemongrass, ginger and chile paste all contribute to the bright, clean and somewhat citrusy aromas and flavors in this Thai-inspired chicken noodle soup. This is the soup for when you feel cold, heavy and weighed down. It clears the sinuses, stimulates damp, boggy tissues and encourages good blood flow.

I personally love using coconut milk to add some creaminess to the soup. It lends a slight tropical note which is so welcome when you are feeling down-and-out with the common cold!

THAI CHICKEN NOODLE SOUP

Flavor Profile: *Pungent, Salty*

Serves: *4 to 6*

1 tbsp (15 ml) melted coconut oil

3–5 cloves garlic, minced

2 tbsp (12 g) minced fresh ginger root

1 tbsp (16 g) chile garlic paste

2 stalks lemongrass, pounded (see Herbalist Tip)

6 cups (1.4 L) Bone Broth with Bone-Building Herbs (page 148) or chicken broth

2 large boneless, skinless chicken breasts

1 cup (130 g) julienned carrots

½ cup (50 g) halved snow peas

1 red bell pepper, julienned

1 (8-oz [226-g]) package brown rice noodles

1 (13.5-oz [398-ml]) can full-fat unsweetened coconut milk

Juice and zest of 1 lime

⅓ cup (6 g) chopped fresh cilantro

½ cup (25 g) bias-cut scallions

1 lime, wedged, for serving

In a large stockpot over medium heat, warm the coconut oil. Sauté the garlic and ginger until fragrant, about 1 to 2 minutes. Add the chile paste, lemongrass, broth and chicken breasts to the pan. Cover and cook it until the chicken is completely cooked through, about 20 minutes.

Turn off the heat and remove the chicken breasts to a cutting board to cool briefly. When the chicken has cooled enough to handle, shred it well with two forks. Strain the stock through a layer or two of cheesecloth; this makes for a really nice clear broth.

Return the broth and the chicken to the stockpot over medium heat. Add the carrots, snow peas and red bell pepper. Increase the heat to medium-high and add the noodles. Cook until the noodles are tender, about 10 minutes or as indicated by the package. Remove the pan from the heat. Stir in the coconut milk.

Add the lime juice and zest, cilantro and scallions. Stir to combine them, ladle the soup into bowls and serve with lime wedges.

Herbalist Tip
To get the most out of your lemongrass, slice the stalk lengthwise and pound lightly with a mallet to help release its aromatic compounds.

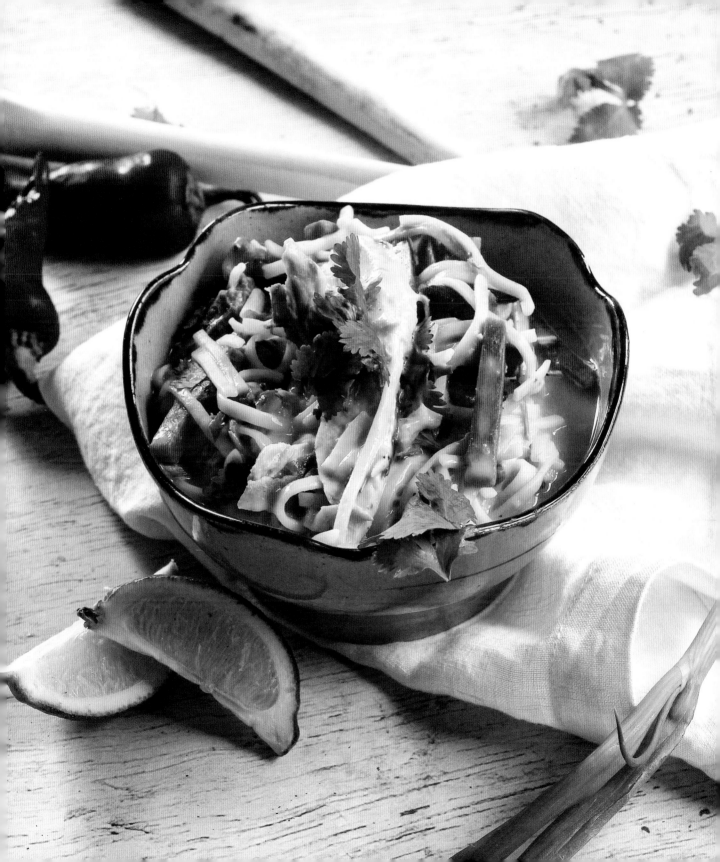

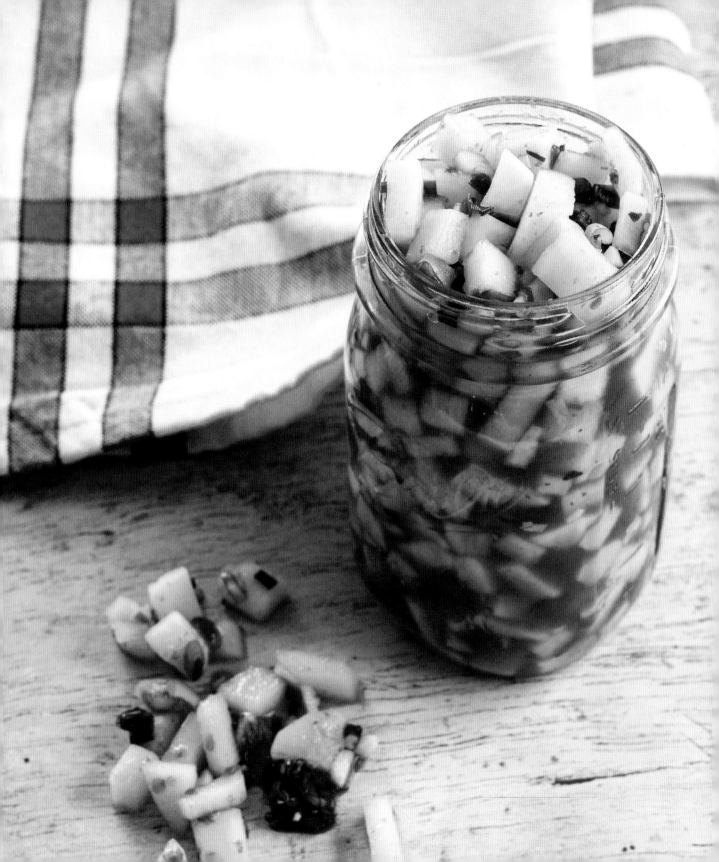

When I decided to write this book, I knew I would include a recipe for kimchi, a popular Korean fermented food. I reached out to my dear friend Ann, of AFarmGirlInTheMaking.com and the *Farm Girl's Guide to Preserving the Harvest*, for ideas and inspiration. Ann is an expert on food preservation and out of her brilliant list of kimchi variations, I immediately lit on her daikon suggestion. Radishes are known for their intense, peppery bite and pungent flavor, but daikon radishes are much milder and slightly sweeter. Daikon are full of vitamin C and possess mild vasodilators that can be helpful for clearing headaches and opening congested, restricted airways. This kimchi is a perfect recipe to foster immunity and good health.

Daikon is traditionally diced for serving as a side dish, or julienned when served as a condiment. This quick fermentation can be ready to eat in as little as 48 hours. I love this kimchi on top of rice or mixed into scrambled eggs!

DAIKON RADISH KIMCHI

Flavor Profile: *Sour, Pungent*

Makes: *2 quarts (1.9 L)*

4 lb (1.8 kg) daikon radish

2 tbsp (34 g) sea salt

2 tbsp (25 g) sugar

¼ cup (60 ml) fish or soy sauce

⅔ cup (160 g) red pepper powder (gochugaru), or to taste

5 scallions, cut into 1-inch (2.5-cm) pieces (optional)

2–3 cloves garlic, minced

Distilled water, as needed

Peel and dice the daikon into ¼-inch (6-mm) cubes or a 1- to 1½-inch (2.5- to 3.5-cm) julienne. Rinse well and pat it dry. Place the daikon in a large bowl and toss it with the salt and sugar until it's well distributed. Cover the bowl with a clean dish cloth and set aside. After 1 hour, drain the daikon, reserving one-quarter of the exuded liquid. Toss the daikon with the fish sauce, reserved liquid, red pepper powder, scallions, if using, and garlic.

Pack this tightly into a ½-gallon (1.9-L) jar, leaving at least 2 inches (5 cm) of headspace to allow for expansion. Liquid should exude to cover the contents within a couple of hours. If the contents of the kimchi are not covered within 2 hours, add just enough distilled water to cover.

Using an airlock lid or a loosely secured plastic lid, ferment the kimchi at room temperature for 48 to 72 hours, tasting regularly after 48 hours for personal preference. The kimchi will become increasingly sour after 72 hours, so it is a matter of flavor preference.

After fermentation, refrigerate the kimchi to slow/stop the fermentation. Refrigerate for 2 to 3 weeks.

Herbalist Tip

Gochugaru is available at most Asian markets and through online retailers. The amount of gochugaru called for in this recipe will result in a moderately intense spice; adjust according to your personal taste.

Cranberries are a classic example of how food serves as medicine. We've all heard cranberry juice suggested for bladder complaints, such as urinary tract infections. But, my friends, store-bought cranberry juice often just isn't the best answer because of the added sugar. If you are down to drinking a few shots of tart cranberry juice to relieve urinary tract discomfort, more power to you. But this spicy, tangy, fruity salsa is a perfect treat. It also brings even more medicinal benefits, including ginger which is traditionally used by herbalists for pelvic complaints. The yogurt whey is optional; some fermentation purists argue that it is unnecessary, but I personally like the results.

Serve this salsa with corn chips or over grilled chicken, pork or even *labneh*—a cheese made from strained yogurt—or with cream cheese.

FERMENTED CRANBERRY SALSA

Flavor Profile: *Sour, Pungent*
Makes: *1 generous pint (about 500 g)*

1 (12-oz [340-g]) package fresh cranberries

1–3 jalapeños, minced

2 tbsp (12 g) finely grated fresh ginger

2 tbsp (28 ml) fresh lime juice

Zest of 1 lime

¼ cup (60 ml) whey drained from organic yogurt (optional)

½ cup (170 g) raw honey

100% cranberry juice or distilled water, as needed to cover

¼ cup (12 g) sliced scallions

¼ cup (4 g) fresh cilantro leaves, minced

Sea salt, to taste

In a food processor, pulse the cranberries until they are well minced. Transfer the cranberries into a medium-sized bowl. Add the jalapeños, ginger, lime juice and zest, whey, if using, and honey. Mix thoroughly. Pack the mixture firmly into a quart-sized (940-ml) glass jar. After a few hours, the juice should cover the mixture; if there is not enough juice, add cranberry juice to cover. Cover the jar with several layers of cheesecloth secured with a rubber band, or with an airlock lid.

Ferment the salsa at room temperature for 7 to 10 days, tasting after about 5 days for preference. When you are satisfied with the fermentation, mix in the scallions, cilantro and sea salt to taste. Serve immediately or store it in the refrigerator for up to 1 week.

Herbalist Tips
I like to add the scallions and cilantro just before serving to add freshness to the fermented salsa.

To gather the whey used in this recipe, drain plain, unflavored yogurt in a fine-mesh sieve lined with muslin or cheesecloth, over a bowl. The whey collected in the bowl is an excellent source of lactic acid bacteria which promote fermentation. The thickened yogurt can be used as Greek yogurt or drained further for a cream cheese–like consistency. This process can take anywhere from 4 to 12 hours, depending on the desired consistency.

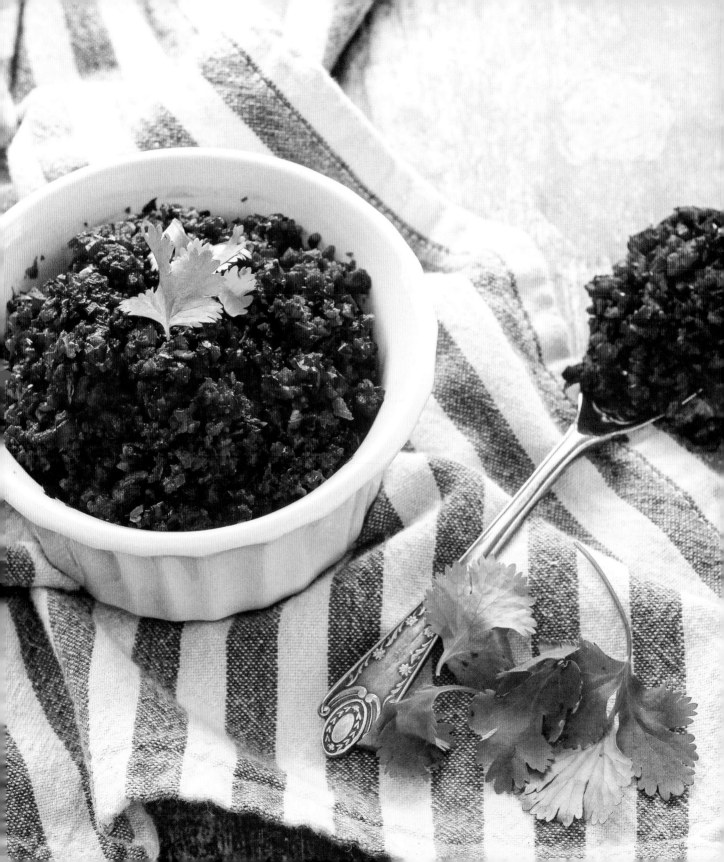

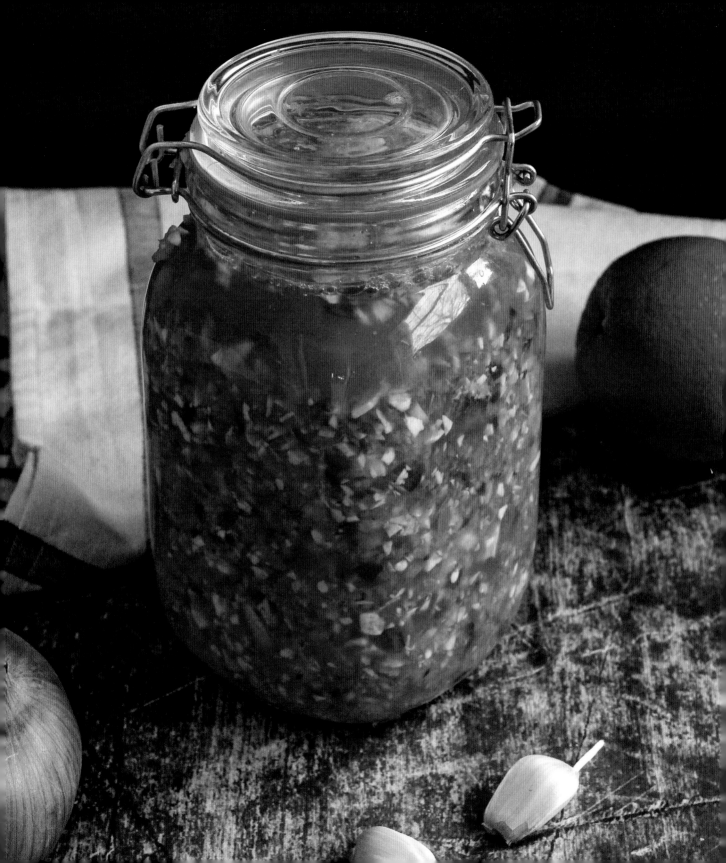

There is perhaps no greater example of a food-based remedy than the classic Fire Cider. This traditional concoction of pungent herbs, roots and vegetables was popularized by the godmother of western herbalism, Rosemary Gladstar. Although this spicy infusion has been met with significant controversy over the years due to the term "fire cider" being trademarked by an unscrupulous brand, it remains one of the most beloved preparations in the standard herbalist repertoire.

A traditional combination of horseradish, onion, garlic, citrus and peppers is boosted with fresh turmeric and black pepper, then infused into raw apple cider vinegar and sweetened with honey. This bold and punchy infusion can be dosed daily as a cold preventative or at the onset of congestion or runny nose. Or it can be used to dress salads, or splashed into braised greens or long-simmered stews to bring flavors alive.

FIRE CIDER

Flavor Profile: *Sour, Pungent*
Makes: *About ½ gallon (1.9 L)*

½ cup (48 g) grated fresh ginger root

½ cup (48 g) grated fresh horseradish root

1 head garlic, minced

1 medium onion, finely chopped

1 jalapeño pepper, sliced

1 orange, peeled and slightly pureed in food processor or thinly sliced

¼ cup (25 g) chopped fresh turmeric root

2 tbsp (16 g) whole black peppercorns

4 cups (940 ml) raw apple cider vinegar (or more to cover)

½–1 cup (170–340 g) raw honey, to taste

Place the ginger, horseradish, garlic, onion, jalapeño, orange, turmeric and peppercorns in a jar. Pour the vinegar over the ingredients to cover them.

If using a metal lid, place a square of wax or parchment paper between the lid and jar. Secure the lid to the jar and infuse it in a dark, cool place, shaking daily for 4 to 6 weeks. Note: The inclusion of turmeric will cause this infusion to stain—clean up any spills promptly.

After the infusion is complete (after 4 to 6 weeks), strain it and add the honey to taste. Bottle and store it in a cool, dark place or in the refrigerator. I bottle my fire cider in 16-ounce glass swing top bottles, giving some as gifts.

Adults may take 1 tablespoon (15 ml) daily, straight or in juice or water as a tonic. Or take 1 tablespoon (15 ml) every 3 to 4 hours for acute cold/flu symptoms.

Children aged 2 to 12 may take 1 teaspoon daily as a tonic in juice or water. Or take ½ teaspoon every 3 to 4 hours for acute symptoms.

Herbalist Tip
After straining out the "marc," or solids, don't throw these pungent tidbits away. You can freeze the spent marc in ice cube trays, or dehydrate it and grind it into a powder. Either form makes an excellent seasoning base for soups, beans and braised dishes!

For me, a week without onions is a week without soul. Maybe that is the reason that I rarely get sick. Onions truly are a magical ingredient. They bring flavor to every dish they grace, and they add health benefits such as antihistamine and antioxidant actions. Thyme offers an intense woodsy flavor to this warming soup as well as a strong antiviral and antimicrobial action—perfect for when cold symptoms hit.

My least favorite task is the time is takes to caramelize onions. Who really has time to stand at the stove for 30 minutes or more waiting for onions to brown, anyway? Use a slow cooker and let time and the appliance do all the work while you go about your day. I like to slice the onions at night and refrigerate them. In the morning, I toss them with melted butter or olive oil, add them to a slow cooker, put on the lid and walk away. Come mealtime, you can transfer the onions to a stockpot, add the rest of the ingredients, garnish and serve. This recipe makes a soup positively teaming with strands of sweet caramelized onions!

SLOW-COOKER FRENCH ONION SOUP WITH THYME

Flavor Profile: *Pungent, Salty*

Serves: *6 as an appetizer or side or 4 as a meal*

4 lb (1.8 kg) yellow onions, sliced pole to pole (about 8–10 cups sliced)

4 tbsp (56 g) butter or olive oil, divided

2 tbsp (16 g) all-purpose flour

1 tbsp (15 ml) Cognac (optional)

1 cup (235 ml) dry white wine

8 cups (1.9 L) Bone Broth with Bone-Building Herbs (page 148) or store-bought beef or chicken broth

3 tbsp (9 g) fresh thyme

4 cups (140 g) 1-inch (2.5-cm) crusty bread cubes, for serving

1 cup (110 g) shredded Gruyère cheese, for serving

Toss the onions and 1 tablespoon (14 g) of butter in a slow cooker. Set the heat to low and place the lid on the slow cooker. Cook for about 10 hours, stirring on occasion if you can. I do not recommend trying to speed up this process by using high heat because it may lead to uneven caramelization.

When the onions are cooked, transfer them to a large stockpot over medium heat. Add 1 tablespoon (14 g) of butter and the flour. Stir well, cooking for 1 to 2 minutes to brown the flour. Raise the heat to medium-high. Add the Cognac, if using, and white wine, and cook for 3 to 4 minutes until the alcohol is mostly cooked off. Add the bone broth and thyme and bring it to a low boil. Reduce the heat to medium-low and place a lid on the soup.

Preheat your oven to 400°F (200°C, or gas mark 6). Melt the remaining 2 tablespoons (28 g) of butter and toss with the bread cubes. Place the bread on a baking sheet and toast it in the oven for 15 to 20 minutes, tossing it occasionally to ensure even browning. When golden and crispy, remove the bread from the oven. Preheat your broiler and place a rack close to the heating element.

To serve, ladle the soup into ovenproof bowls. Top them with bread cubes and cheese. Place the bowls under the broiler until the cheese is melted, bubbly and slightly browned, about 1 to 2 minutes. Serve immediately.

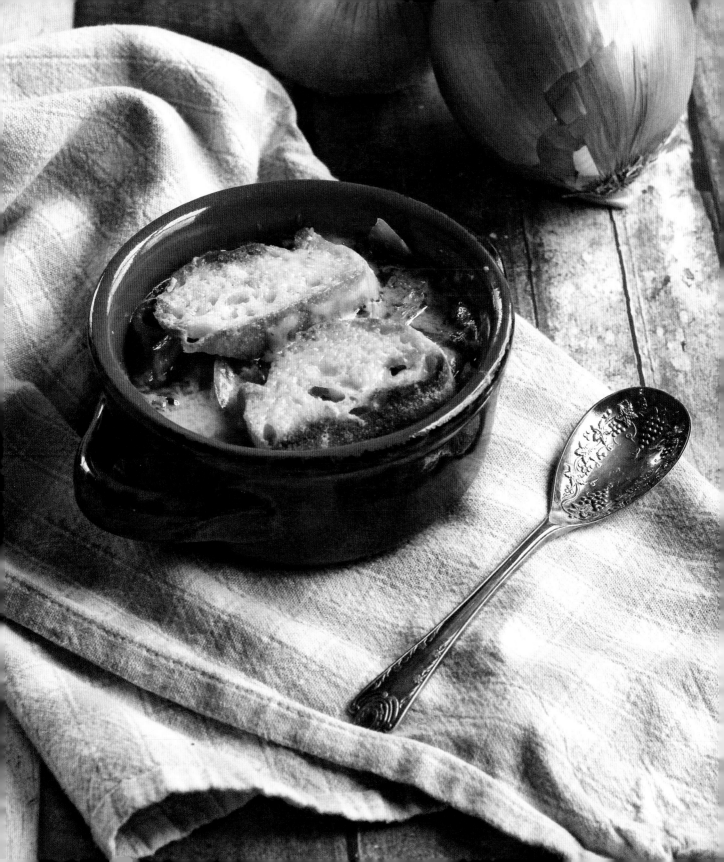

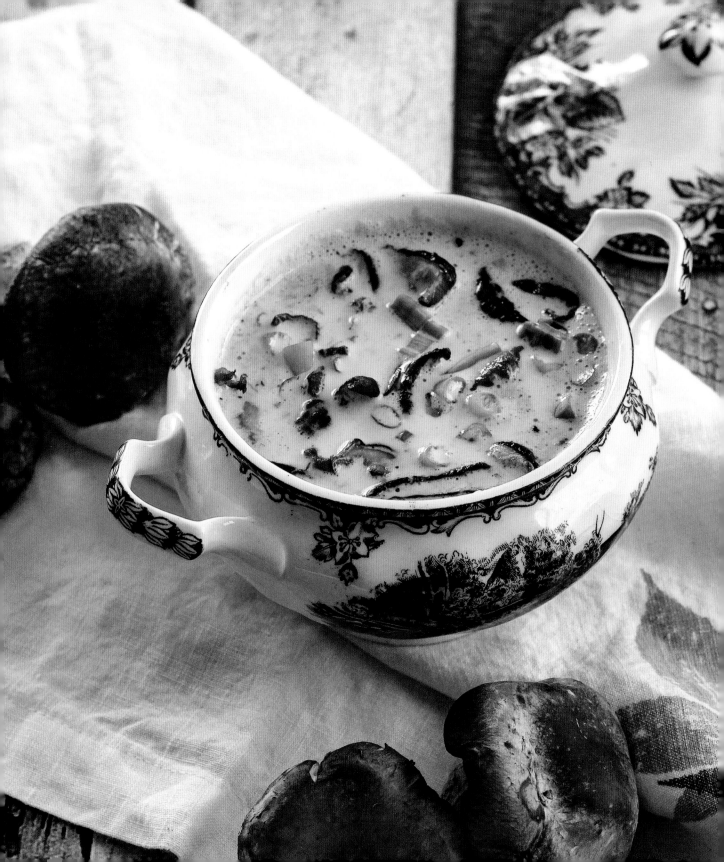

When we consider herbs and foods for immunity, we often think in terms of acute needs. We reach for what I refer to as the emergency herbs and foods—namely pungent, spicy, often sinus-clearing selections such as garlic, horseradish and ginger.

There is another aspect of immunity that so often goes ignored. Shiitake mushrooms are an immune modulator—they zero in on an imbalanced immune system. This is of key importance to those facing acute illness and those with chronic autoimmune issues. While long-term use of shiitakes or any other immunomodulator should be discussed with your physician, a creamy shiitake soup is an excellent way to promote good health. This earthy soup is as wholesome as it is delicious.

CREAMY WHOLESOME SHIITAKE SOUP

Flavor Profile: *Sweet, Salty*

Serves: *4 to 6*

16 oz (454 g) large, whole shiitake mushrooms

2 cups (320 g) finely chopped onion

1 cup (130 g) finely chopped carrot

2 tbsp (28 g) butter, melted

2–3 cloves garlic, minced

2½ cups (590 ml) water

2 tbsp (12 g) shiitake powder

1 tbsp (3 g) fresh thyme leaves (or 1 tsp dried)

1½ cups (355 ml) half-and-half

⅓ cup (16 g) sliced scallions

De-stem and slice the shiitakes into ⅛-inch (3-mm) slices. Set them aside.

In a large stockpot over medium heat, sweat the onion and carrot in the melted butter until the onions are translucent, about 7 to 10 minutes, stirring frequently. Add the garlic and shiitakes, then cook 3 to 5 minutes until the shiitakes start to tenderize, stirring gently.

Remove about one-third of the mushroom mixture and puree it in a blender until smooth. Add the puree back to the pot with the water, shiitake powder and thyme. Cover the pot and simmer over medium-low heat for about 20 minutes. After cooking, remove it from the heat. Stir in the half-and-half and add the scallions. Ladle the soup into bowls.

Herbalist Tip

Make your own shiitake powder by grinding dried shiitakes to a fine powder in a spice grinder.

Sunny, fragrant Meyer lemons are a perfect wintertime treat in the northern hemisphere. And what serendipitous timing, given that winter is a time when seasonal viruses run rampant. Lemons are a fantastic source of vitamin C, which helps to protect the immune system. Bay leaves are another source of vitamin C and are reputed to soothe bodily aches and pains.

Salt-preserved lemon is absolutely delicious. Add the sliced rind to tapenades and compound butters, or use it to brighten long-braised or roasted dishes. Try these in the Mediterranean Olive Salad with Israeli Couscous (page 86) or simply slice a few bits into your favorite chicken noodle soup.

Pick organic, spray- and wax-free Meyer lemons for this recipe. The amount of lemons needed to fill each quart-sized (940-ml) jar may differ due to the size of the lemons. I find that six usually pack the jar well and cover the flesh with the citrusy, salty brine.

SALT-PRESERVED MEYER LEMONS WITH BAY LEAVES

Flavor Profile: *Sour, Salty, Bitter*

Makes: *About 1 quart (663 g)*

4–6 organic, spray- and wax-free Meyer lemons

1 tbsp (15 g) sea salt, plus ½ tbsp (about 8 g) per lemon

2–3 bay leaves, fresh or dry

Additional fresh lemon juice, if needed

Wash and rinse the lemons well. Slice the lemons lengthwise three times, leaving about ½ inch (1.3 cm) of one end intact so that the lemon is divided into six even segments.

Place 1 tablespoon (15 g) of sea salt in the bottom of a clean quart-sized (940-ml) jar. Over the mouth of the jar, sprinkle ½ tablespoon (8 g) of salt into the cavity of each lemon. Repeat with each lemon segment, stuffing the jar firmly with enough force to see the lemons start to give off their juice. Push bay leaves down the sides of the jar until they're completely covered. Cover with a tight-fitting lid and set it aside for 24 hours.

After 24 hours, the brine created by the citrus juice and salt should cover the lemons completely. If the lemons are not submerged, mash them down a little more or add enough fresh lemon juice to cover them.

Allow the lemons and bay leaves to brine for 2 to 3 weeks. When the rinds are soft and chewy, the reserved lemons can be stored in the refrigerator for up to 6 months. Be sure to keep the lemons submerged at all times to prevent mold growth.

Herbalist Tip

We are after the rind with these preserved lemons; much, if not all, of the pulp will disintegrate during the brining and fermentation process. To use, remove the needed amount of preserved lemons from the jar and rinse them well. Chop, slice or mince them as your recipe calls for, or as desired.

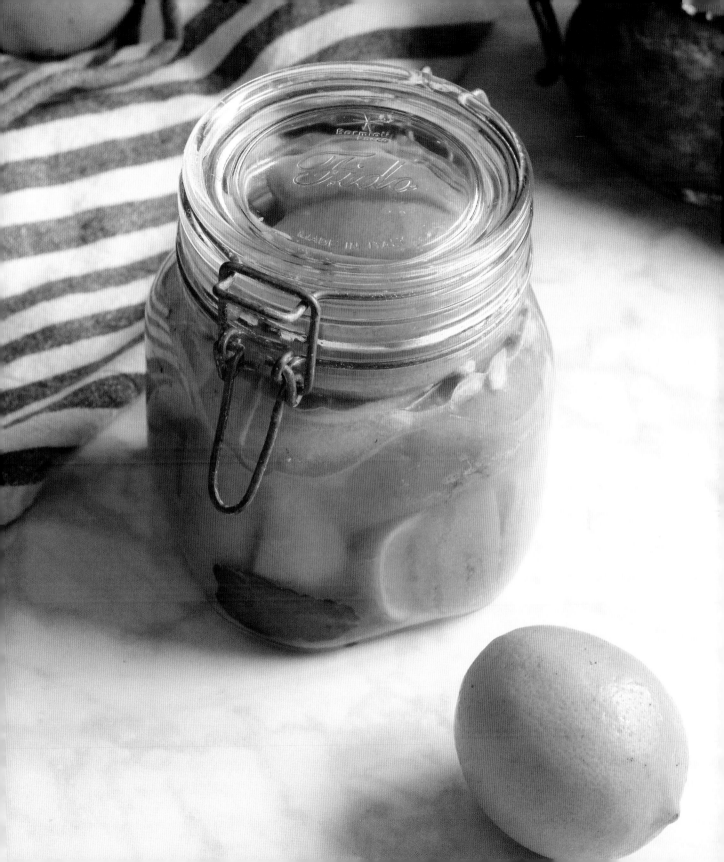

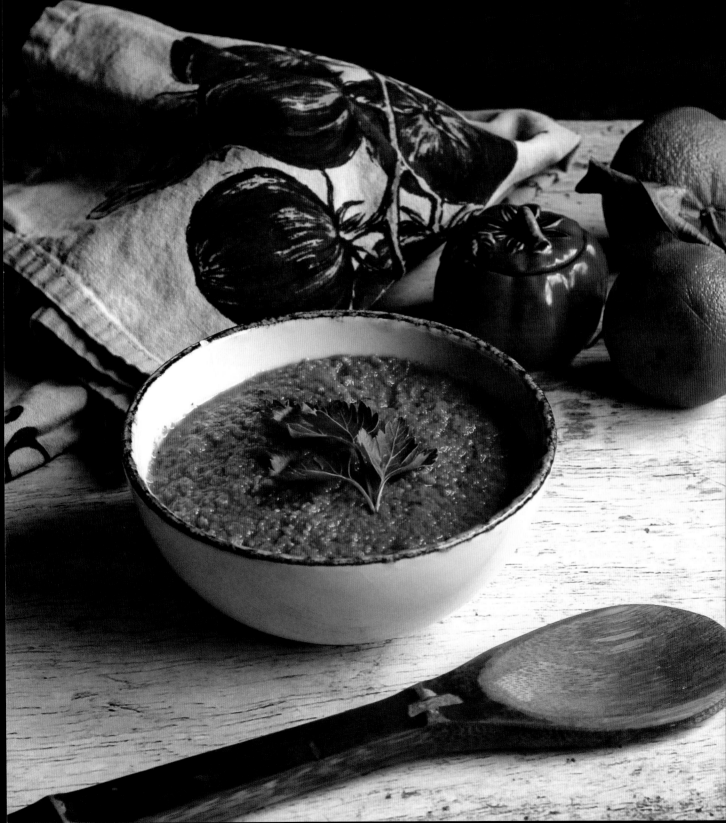

Tomatoes and oranges. You read that right. The first time I was invited to taste a soup like this my eyebrows raised with skepticism, too. But it is oh-my-goodness good.

Sour flavors are a great indicator of foods that have some serious immune-boosting muscle. Tomatoes and oranges are both high in vitamin C, offering excellent antioxidant action, protecting and repairing our cells. This is a soup to make when flu season hits your workplace or your child's classroom. It is the culinary version of a "no trespassing" sign, protecting the immune system.

While other recipes use just juice, I blend the whole orange to get all the health benefits of the peel and pith into the soup. Choose a low-pith orange, such as a navel or cara cara. I like to use home-canned tomatoes, but store-bought diced or crushed tomatoes will work fine. Adding cumin and coriander brings depth of flavor while fortifying the immune-boosting nature of this meal. This simple soup is an ideal weeknight meal that is frugal, medicinal and delicious!

TOMATO-ORANGE SOUP

Flavor Profile: *Sour, Bitter*

Serves: *4 to 6*

1 large or 2 small oranges

2 tbsp (30 ml) extra-virgin olive oil

½ yellow onion, diced

2–3 cloves garlic, minced

1 tbsp (16 g) tomato paste

½ tsp cumin

1 tsp ground coriander

1 (28-oz [794-g]) can diced or crushed tomatoes

¼ tsp baking soda

½ cup (120 ml) heavy cream

Salt & freshly ground pepper, to taste

Parsley, for garnish (optional)

Toasted baguette, for serving

Cut the orange into halves or quarters. In a food processor, puree the orange to a fine, mealy pulp, about 1 minute, scraping down the sides as needed.

In a large saucepan over medium heat, add the oil and onion. Sauté until the onion is translucent, about 5 to 7 minutes, stirring frequently. Add the garlic, tomato paste, cumin and coriander. Stir well and continue cooking until it's fragrant, about 2 minutes.

Add the diced tomatoes, baking soda and pureed orange and reduce the heat to medium-low. Cover and cook for 15 to 20 minutes, stirring occasionally.

After cooking, remove the pan from the heat. Blend it to a smooth puree in a blender or food processor, or using an immersion blender. Stir in the heavy cream and season with salt and pepper to taste. Garnish with parsley, if using, and serve with a crusty baguette.

Nothing wakes you up like wasabi! Energetically speaking, wasabi is downright hot and dry, and produces a strong salivary response. It's an excellent quick remedy for a stuffed-up head.

This pungent root is a favorite condiment on sushi, but wasabi almonds are becoming a favorite offering in the snack food aisle. They are so easy to make at home, and they taste a million times better. You can certainly adjust the wasabi to your preferred level of heat. Remember, the fierier these almonds are the quicker you'll be breathing clearly again—maybe breathing fire, but at least you'll be breathing!

WAKE-UP WASABI ALMONDS

Flavor Profile: *Sour, Sweet, Pungent*

Makes: *4 cups (580 g)*

1 egg white

1 tbsp (15 ml) coconut aminos or soy sauce

1–3 tbsp (6–18 g) wasabi powder

2 tsp (6 g) cornstarch

4 cups (580 g) whole raw almonds

Preheat your oven to 300°F (150°C, or gas mark 2). In a medium-sized bowl, whisk the egg white just until frothy. Mix it with the coconut aminos, wasabi powder and cornstarch. Add the almonds and toss well to coat them.

Bake the almonds on a lined sheet pan for about 30 minutes, stirring occasionally. After baking, remove them from the oven and cool completely before storing in an airtight container.

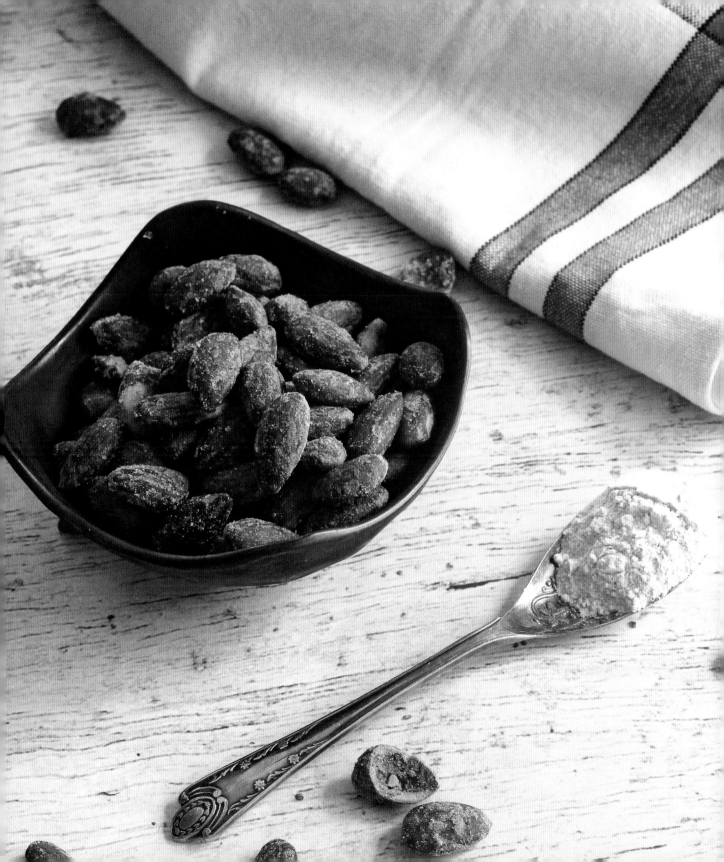

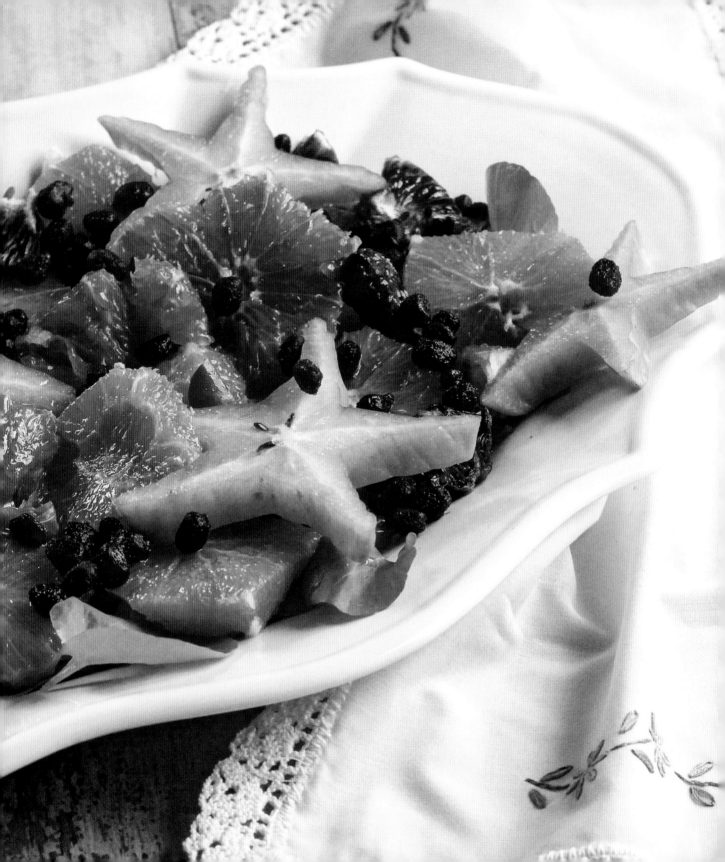

Oranges and other citrus-family fruits have a long-standing reputation for fighting the common cold and helping you maintain excellent wellness. Full of sour and powerful antioxidants, these fruits can muscle away a cold before it even starts.

This salad is complemented with festive slices of star fruit and studded with jewel-like pomegranate seeds. Mixed with peppery, sinus-opening watercress, this salad is lovely atop a steak cut of an oil-rich fish, such as swordfish, albacore or salmon.

I particularly love the inclusion of pomegranate molasses in the dressing, though honey is an acceptable substitute.

SAVORY CITRUS SALAD

Flavor Profile: *Sour*

Serves: *4 to 6*

2 medium oranges, peeled and sliced into ¼-inch (6-mm)-thick rounds

3 medium blood oranges, peeled and sliced into ¼-inch (6-mm)-thick rounds

2 medium pink grapefruit, peeled and sliced into ¼-inch (6-mm)-thick rounds

2 medium star fruit, sliced ¼ inch (6 mm) thick

1 cup (175 g) pomegranate seeds

1 bunch watercress, rinsed and stems chopped off

2 tbsp (30 ml) red wine vinegar

1 tbsp (15 ml) pomegranate molasses or honey

¼ cup (60 ml) extra-virgin olive oil

Pinch of salt, or to taste

Grilled fish or chicken, for serving

Toss the oranges, grapefruit, star fruit, pomegranate seeds and watercress in a large bowl.

Prepare the dressing by combining the vinegar and pomegranate molasses in a small bowl. Slowly whisk in the olive oil until it's emulsified, about 30 seconds. Season with salt to taste. Gently toss the fruit and watercress with the dressing.

Serve the salad on its own or over grilled fish or chicken.

While shiitakes, lion's mane and turkey tail mushrooms get all the medicinal credit, simple cremini mushrooms are full of nutrition and powerful immune-modulating phytonutrients. Miso acts as an umami-rich flavor agent in this recipe, and it is full of its own health benefits. As a probiotic fermented soy product, miso is associated with improved gut health and immune function.

These mushrooms are the perfect side dish to a roasted bird, steak or fillet of salmon. They also make a tasty vegetarian meal served over a bed of rice. Garnish with chopped flat-leaf parsley and scallions.

CREMINI MUSHROOMS WITH MISO BUTTER

Flavor Profile: *Salty, Sweet*
Serves: *4 to 6 as a side dish*

1 tbsp (15 ml) extra-virgin olive oil

2 lb (900 g) cremini mushrooms, halved if especially large

¼ cup (56 g) softened butter

2 tbsp (32 g) miso paste (I prefer a yellow or other mild miso paste.)

2–3 cloves garlic, minced

2 scallions, cut on the diagonal

¼ cup (15 g) chopped flat-leaf parsley (optional)

In a skillet over medium-high heat, add the oil and mushrooms. Sauté until the mushrooms are brown, stirring frequently, about 10 to 15 minutes.

Prepare the miso butter by combining the butter, miso and garlic, stirring well.

When the mushrooms are browned, turn the heat to low. Add the miso butter and cook for 2 to 3 minutes, until the garlic is fragrant.

Remove the skillet from the heat. Toss the mushrooms with the parsley and scallions, and serve warm.

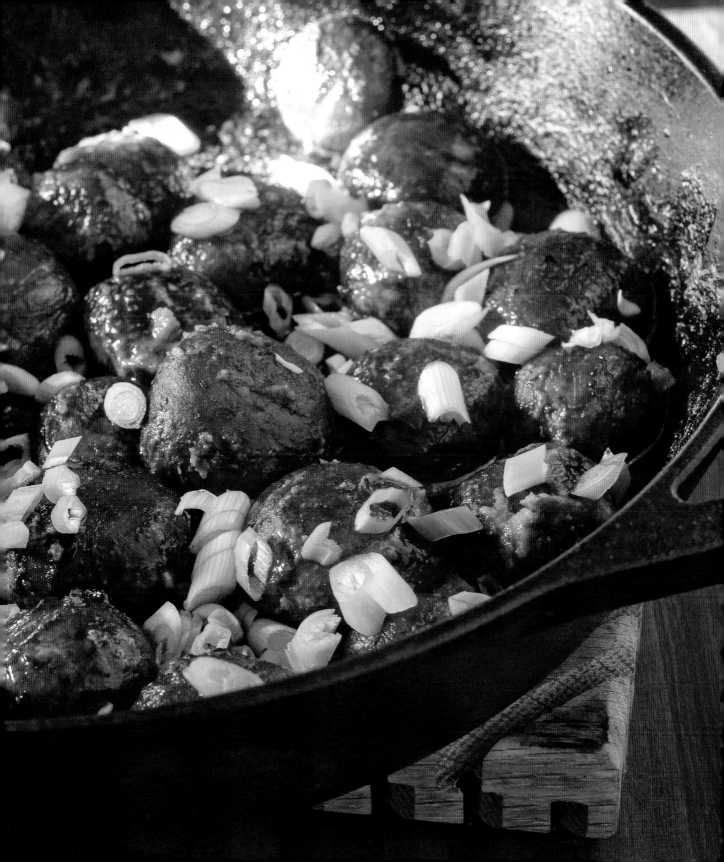

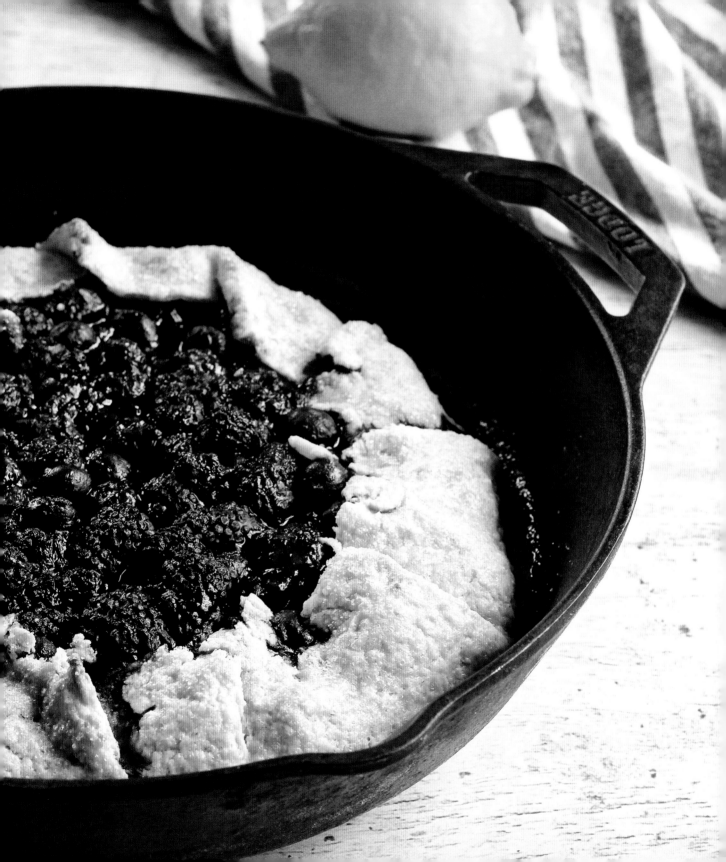

FOUR

RECIPES TO

INVIGORATE YOUR CARDIOVASCULAR HEALTH

The ole ticker and its associated organs get a lot of attention. Cardiovascular disease is still the leading cause of death for men and women in the United States—accounting for roughly twenty-five percent of deaths each year. Startling statistics, no?

When we refer to cardiovascular health, it is more than the heart organ. We mean the complex network of blood vessels—capillaries, veins and arteries. This network must always work at peak performance or we quickly become sick. So how do we maintain this essential system?

Cardiovascular health is complex, as are the food choices that we make to support its well-being. Pungent herbs such as garlic and cayenne have diffusive benefits that help to clear blockages. The antioxidant actions of cocoa and hawthorn protect fragile cardiovascular tissues from free radicals.

Garlic lovers will swoon and hearts will soar with Chicken with 50 Garlic Cloves (page 82). Or try the healthy fats and herbal properties of Fennel-Encrusted Salmon (page 93) to help reduce damaging inflammation. And for the occasional indulgence, I have a treat for you with my Chocolate & Hawthorne Berry Flourless Torte (page 98)!

Your heart and vessels serve you well. Now give them all the love they deserve—and care for them deliciously.

This classic recipe hits all the marks for flavor and good health: pungent roasted garlic and warm, woodsy thyme combine with satiny bone broth, tender chicken thighs and a subtle acidity from white wine and verjus. Together they create a dish that deeply nourishes the cardiovascular system. Garlic is renowned as one of the world's most robust antioxidants, and it has demonstrated an ability to help maintain healthy cholesterol levels. Thyme is an earthy herb that also promotes healthy blood pressure and lipid profiles. Serve this dish with a side of sautéed bitter greens and a grilled baguette to mop up the glorious juices.

CHICKEN WITH 50 GARLIC CLOVES

Flavor Profile: *Pungent*

Serves: *4 to 6*

3 whole heads garlic

1 cut-up whole chicken (breast split in two horizontally)

Sea salt & freshly ground pepper, to taste

2 tbsp (28 g) butter

1 tbsp (15 ml) extra-virgin olive oil

2 tbsp (16 g) all-purpose flour

½ cup (120 ml) dry white wine

¾ cup (175 ml) chicken bone broth

2 tbsp (6 g) fresh thyme leaves

1–2 tbsp (15–30 ml) verjus or champagne vinegar

Baguette, sliced and grilled, for serving

Herbalist Tip

Use a cast-iron skillet to increase the trace mineral content of this meal.

Remove the individual cloves from the heads of garlic. Blanch the garlic cloves in boiling water for 30 seconds, then strain and rinse them under cool water. The papery peels can now be removed easily and discarded. Set the peeled cloves aside.

Trim the fat pockets from the chicken pieces. Season both sides of the chicken liberally with salt and pepper. Preheat your oven to 350°F (175°C, or gas mark 4).

In a large cast-iron or heavy-bottomed skillet over medium heat, melt the butter and add the olive oil. Place the chicken pieces skin-side down in the skillet, working in batches so as not to overcrowd the pan. Cook until the skin is golden and releases easily from the pan, about 5 to 7 minutes, and the remaining fat is well rendered. Flip and cook the other side for 5 minutes. Remove the chicken from the pan and continue this step until all the chicken is seared on both sides. Set the chicken aside on a plate to capture any juices.

In the same pan over medium heat, add the peeled garlic cloves. Sauté the garlic for 7 to 10 minutes, until golden on both sides and fragrant. Add the flour to the garlic and pan juices. Stir them constantly over the heat for 2 minutes to cook off the raw flour flavor; add the white wine slowly while stirring vigorously to break up any clumps of flour and scrape any browned bits from the pan bottom and sides. Add the chicken bone broth and thyme and stir to combine them. Turn off the heat and add the chicken skin-side up and any juices back to the skillet.

Carefully transfer the skillet to the oven. Bake uncovered for about 25 to 30 minutes, or until a meat thermometer registers 165°F (74°C). At this point, you can blast it under a broiler for 2 to 3 minutes to crisp up the skin if you'd like.

When the chicken is done, transfer the skillet back to the stove top. Using tongs, carefully remove the chicken pieces and transfer them to a serving platter with rimmed sides. Return the pan sauce to a simmer over medium heat and add the verjus to taste. Adjust the sauce to your desired consistency by adding more liquid—I prefer to use bone broth—or cooking it down to thicken. Adjust the seasoning to taste.

Serve the chicken with slices of grilled baguette to mop up the delicious juices and roasted garlic-y goodness.

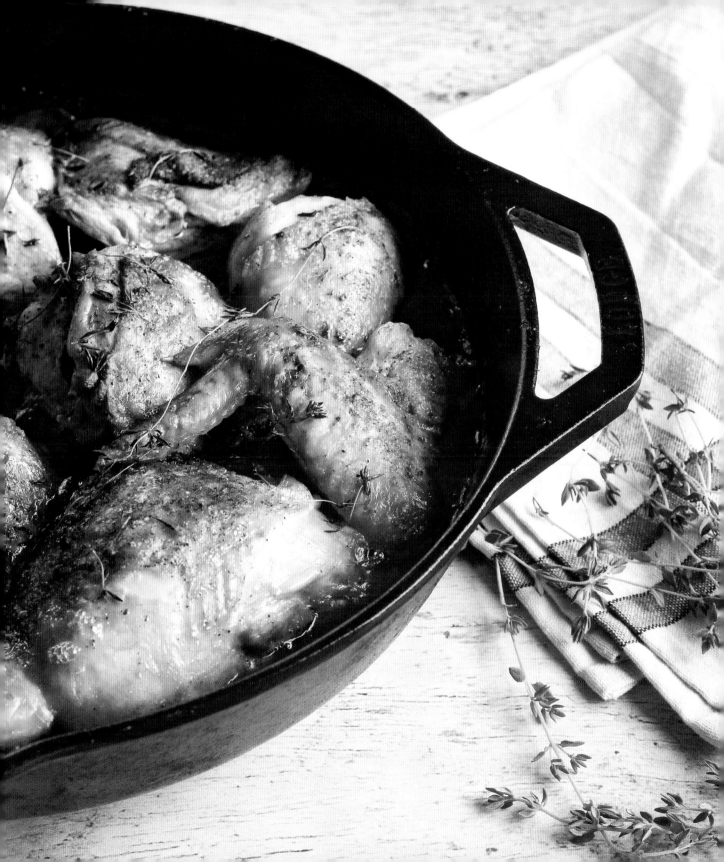

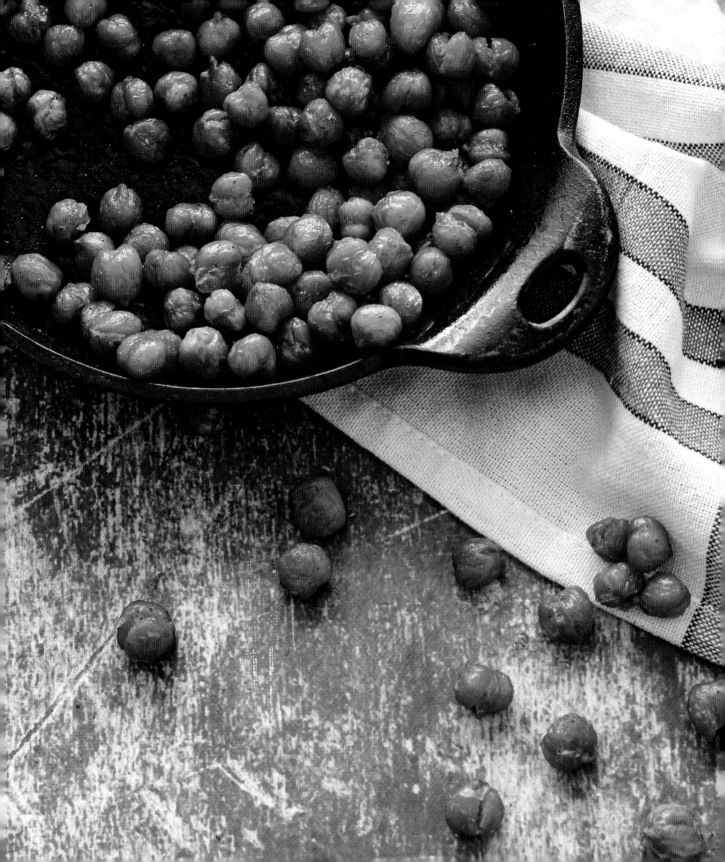

Garbanzo beans, also known as chickpeas, are often relegated to the snack table in the form of creamy hummus. While hummus is a delicious dish, garbanzo beans can be transformed into a spicy little snack that will satiate your taste buds and please your cardiovascular system!

Garbanzo beans are a significant source of fiber, and these beans offer great potential for helping to reduce elevated cholesterol levels and high blood pressure. The fiber also increases your sense of fullness, encourages bowel regularity and promotes healthy gut flora.

This protein- and fiber-rich snack also has the generous addition of cayenne pepper. This warming herb has long been used by herbalists to reduce pain and inflammation. Recent studies indicate that cayenne pepper may help to relax blood vessels and ease high blood pressure.
This spicy snack is a perfect way to introduce heart-healthy fiber and inflammation-reducing spices to your diet!

CAYENNE-ROASTED GARBANZO BEANS

Flavor Profile: *Sweet, Pungent*

Serves: *2 to 4*

1 (15.5-oz [439-g]) can garbanzo beans, drained

2 tbsp (30 ml) extra-virgin olive oil

½ tsp salt (optional)

½ tsp cayenne pepper

½ tsp granulated garlic

¼ tsp ground cumin

Preheat your oven to 450°F (230°C, or gas mark 8). Drain and rinse the garbanzo beans. On a lined baking sheet, mix the beans, olive oil, salt, if using, cayenne pepper, garlic and cumin until the beans are evenly coated. Roast for 35 minutes, until golden and crispy, stirring once halfway through cooking.

As an alternative, roast for 15 minutes for softer beans that are great served over Cilantro-Lime Rice (page 21).

We've all heard of the Mediterranean diet and its health benefits. Wine, fish, fresh vegetables, fruit, aromatic herbs, whole grains—what's not to love?! Olives are at the core of the Mediterranean diet, and they're rich in heart-healthy oils that contain the powerful antioxidant vitamin E and the blood pressure–regulating phytonutrient quercetin.

This salad is positively brimming with flavor, luxurious oils and eye-popping color. I like to choose olives in a variety of colors, including green, black and purple. Rosemary, parsley and preserved lemons also add profound antioxidant action to this already heart-friendly dish!

MEDITERRANEAN OLIVE SALAD WITH ISRAELI COUSCOUS

Flavor Profile: *Salty, Bitter, Pungent*

Serves: *4 to 6*

¼ cup (60 ml) vegetable broth

1 cup (175 g) Israeli couscous

3 cups (weight will vary) assorted, pitted olives, coarsely chopped

1 cup (150 g) roasted red bell peppers, coarsely chopped

1 (6-oz [170-g]) jar marinated artichoke hearts, drained

¼ cup (15 g) flat-leaf parsley, coarsely chopped

1 tbsp (2 g) finely minced fresh rosemary

2 tbsp (45 g) Salt-Preserved Meyer Lemons with Bay Leaves (page 70), or zest of 1 lemon

Dressing

¼ cup (60 ml) red wine vinegar

¼ tsp Dijon mustard

2 cloves garlic, finely minced

¾ cup (175 ml) extra-virgin olive oil

Salt & freshly ground pepper, to taste

¾ cup (4 oz [115 g]) feta cheese, crumbled, for garnish

Prepare the couscous by bringing the broth to a boil over medium-high heat. Add the couscous and return it to a boil, then reduce the heat to medium-low to maintain a gentle simmer. Cook for 10 minutes, until the pearls are al dente— tender throughout but firm to the tooth. Drain and set it aside to cool.

In a medium-sized bowl, toss the olives, roasted peppers, artichoke hearts, parsley, rosemary and lemon rind.

To make the dressing, in a separate bowl, add the red wine vinegar, mustard and garlic, whisking well to combine them. Slowly drizzle in the olive oil, whisking well to emulsify it, about 30 seconds. Season with salt and pepper to taste.

Add the couscous and the dressing to the olive mixture. Toss well to combine them. Garnish with crumbled feta cheese.

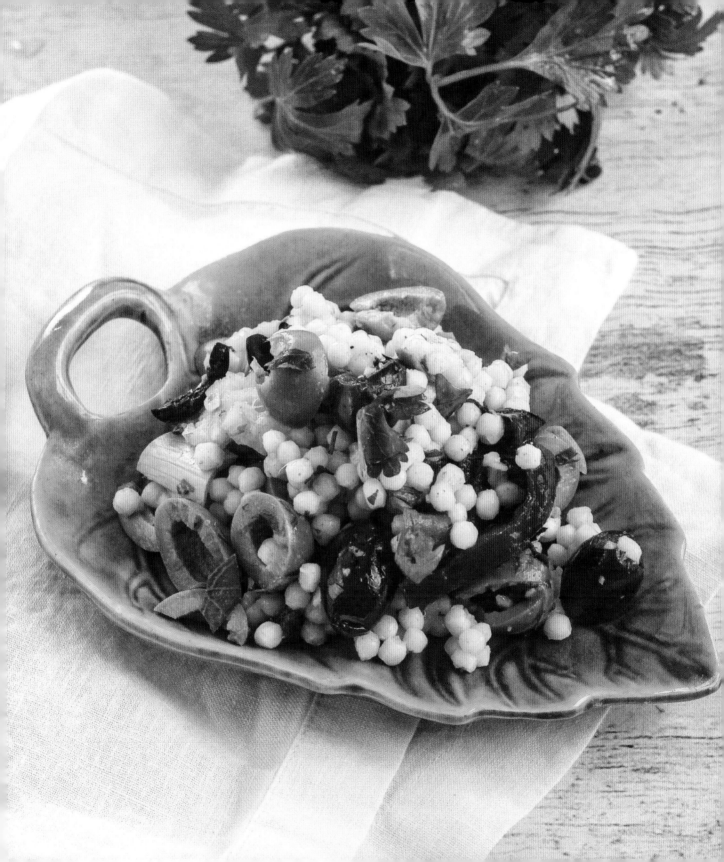

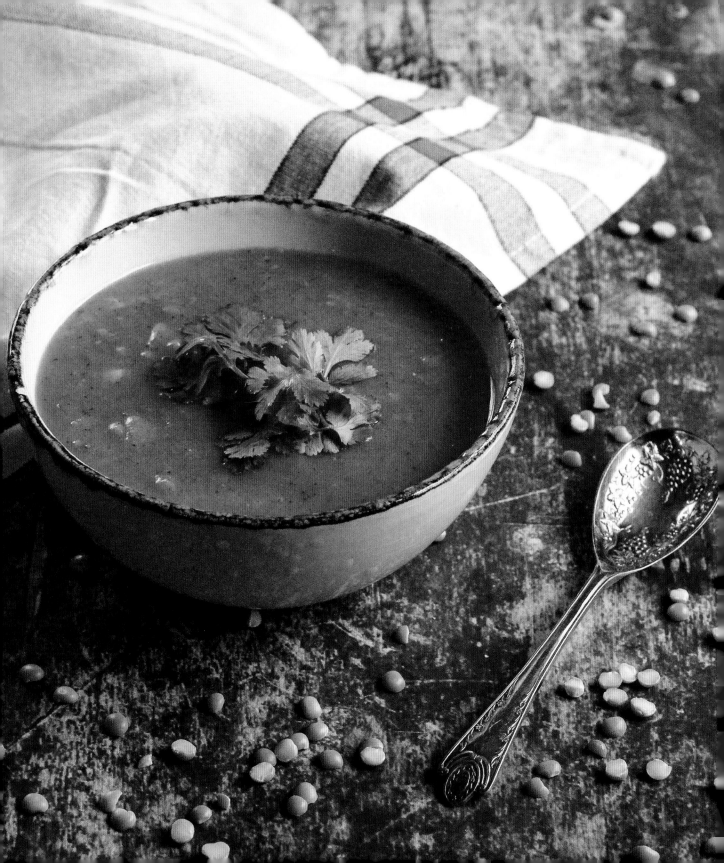

I was first introduced to dal in my very early teen years, and I was struck by the vibrant color and earthy flavor of the soup. It was perhaps my first taste of Indian cooking, and I was hooked. But dal isn't just a tasty meal. It is so much more!

Lentils are fiber-rich and loaded with antioxidants that have profound benefits for the cardiovascular system. They have a high protein content, as well as abundant B vitamins and minerals such as magnesium, potassium and zinc. Several studies indicate anti-inflammatory and antioxidant benefits from lentils. Cumin plays a major role in the flavor of this soup and also seems to improve HDL cholesterol levels.

This soup is perfect for a weeknight dinner, as yellow lentils are already split and cook quite quickly.

YELLOW LENTIL DAL WITH CUMIN

Flavor Profile: *Sweet, Pungent*

Serves: *4*

1 onion, chopped

2 cloves garlic, minced

1 tbsp (15 ml) extra-virgin olive oil

1 tsp ground turmeric

2 tsp (2 g) ground cumin

1½ cups (288 g) yellow lentils

8 cups (1.9 L) Bone Broth with Bone-Building Herbs (page 148) or vegetable broth

2 tbsp (28 ml) fresh lemon juice

Salt & freshly ground pepper, to taste

¼ cup (15 g) flat-leaf parsley, chopped, for garnish

In a stockpot over medium heat, sauté the onion and garlic in olive oil until the onion is soft and translucent, about 5 to 7 minutes, stirring frequently. Add the turmeric and cumin and "bloom" for 1 to 2 minutes, until the spices are aromatic. Add the lentils and broth and bring it to a low boil. Reduce the heat to medium-low and cover the pot.

Cook for 20 to 25 minutes, until the lentils are tender. Remove the dal from the heat. Puree about half of the soup using a blender or an immersion blender. Return it to the pot and stir in the lemon juice. Season with salt and pepper to taste.

Ladle the soup into bowls and garnish with parsley.

Berries, with their sweetness, may seem like a naughty treat, but they are far more virtuous than one might imagine. Berries are ripe with polyphenols and antioxidants that contribute to heart health. They also are associated with reduced cholesterol levels, improved circulation and improved response to oxidative stress! The herb lemon verbena in this galette brings citrusy, floral-lemon notes and imparts its own antioxidant cardiovascular benefits.

I love this simple, rustic tart. Crafted with an almond crust and filled with a jumble of sun-ripened berries, this tart has just the type of casual elegance that I so enjoy.

MIXED SUMMER BERRY GALETTE

Flavor Profile: *Sour, Sweet*

Serves: *6*

Crust

⅓ cup (35 g) sliced almonds

1½ cups (188 g) all-purpose flour

2 tbsp (26 g) sugar

½ tsp salt

½ cup (112 g) cold unsalted butter, cut into pieces

⅓ cup (80 ml) cold water

1 egg yolk, beaten

Berry Filling

2 cups (250 g) fresh raspberries

1 cup (145 g) fresh blueberries

1 cup (145 g) fresh blackberries

¼ cup (50 g) granulated sugar, or to taste

1 tbsp (8 g) all-purpose flour

1 tsp finely grated lemon zest

2 tbsp (12 g) fresh lemon verbena, minced

For the crust, in a food processor, grind the almonds until they are a fine sand-like texture. Add the flour, 1 tablespoon (13 g) sugar and salt and pulse to combine them. Add the butter and pulse until a coarse meal forms. With the food processor running, drizzle in the cold water, stopping when the dough forms a cohesive ball. On a lightly floured surface, pat the dough out into two equal discs. Wrap the discs in plastic film and chill for at least 30 minutes.

Preheat your oven to 400°F (200°C, or gas mark 6). Line a baking sheet or a cast-iron pan with parchment paper.

To make the berry filling, toss the berries, sugar, flour, lemon zest and lemon verbena. Set it aside. Roll the chilled dough into circles about 12 inches (30 cm) across. Transfer the discs to the lined baking sheet. Fill the centers of each disc with the berry mixture and fold the edges of the dough over the fruit. Brush the edges of the dough with the beaten egg yolk and dust them lightly with the remaining 1 tablespoon (13 g) sugar.

Bake for about 40 minutes, or until the crust is golden. After baking, remove the galettes from the oven. Cool them on a wire rack and slice into wedges to serve.

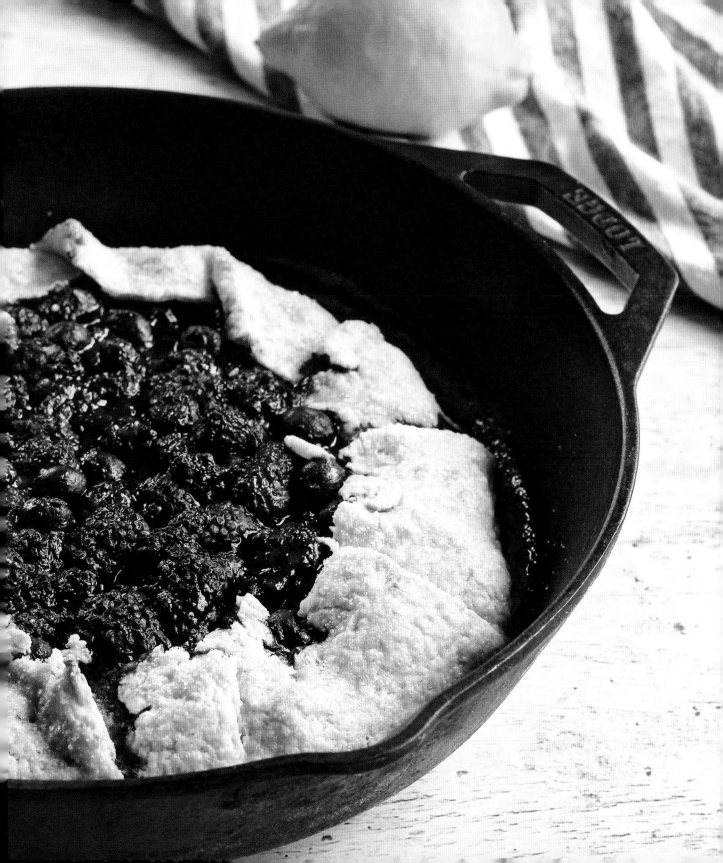

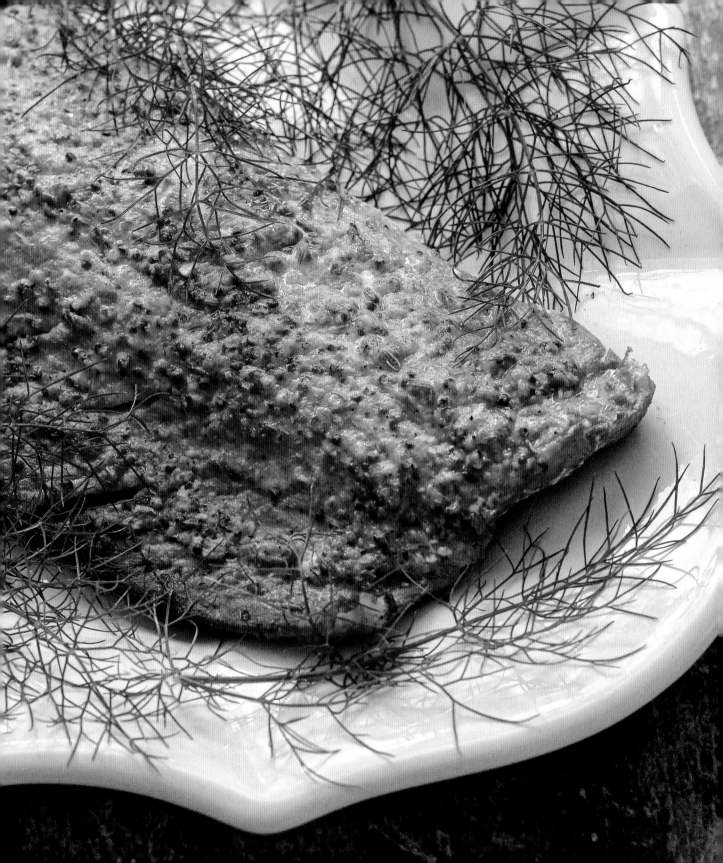

This salmon is food for your taste buds and for your heart. The benefits of salmon are well known: studies indicate that eating one to two servings weekly of fish rich in omega-3 fatty acids may reduce heart disease complaints and the risk of cardiac death.

One of my favorite culinary and medicinal herbs also offers significant heart-health benefits. Licorice-y fennel seeds contain vitamins, minerals and phytonutrients that have a demonstrated positive effect on cholesterol-level reduction and reduction in blood pressure.

I love to serve this salmon with sautéed fennel bulbs for added fennel-y goodness.

FENNEL-ENCRUSTED SALMON

Flavor Profile: *Salty, Sweet, Pungent*

Serves: *4*

2 tbsp (12 g) whole fennel seeds

1½ tsp (4 g) whole peppercorns

1½ tsp (7 g) sea salt

1 tbsp (15 ml) extra-virgin olive oil

3 tbsp (45 g) Dijon mustard

1 lb (450 g) wild-caught salmon fillet

Preheat your oven to 400°F (200°C, or gas mark 6).

In a dedicated spice grinder, or using a mortar and pestle, grind the fennel seeds, peppercorns and sea salt until they resemble a fine powder.

Place a heavy-bottomed pan, ideally cast-iron, over medium heat. Add the oil. While the pan is heating, mix the fennel powder with the mustard and smear it evenly on the flesh side of the salmon fillet. Place the fillet in the pan, skin-side down. Cook for 5 minutes, then transfer the salmon to the oven. Cook for another 5 to 7 minutes, until the fish flakes.

Cut the salmon into individual portions and serve immediately.

Herbalist Tip

This salmon is also delicious cold, served over greens and dressed lightly with a simple vinaigrette.

Chocolate in a savory application is a rarity, but it is perhaps one of the most meaningful ways that we can harness the heart-friendly benefits of this famous treat. Cacao, in the form of chocolate or cocoa, is often used in herbalism for its mood-elevating and heart-health benefits. Bolstered by the invigorating effects of spicy chiles and full-bodied spices, a classic mole sauce is a dish made for cardiovascular health. Pumpkin seeds offer additional fiber and give texture to the sauce. They even impart their own medicinal virtues (see page 14).

I particularly love this mole sauce served over a grilled chicken breast with Cilantro-Lime Rice (page 21). This mole can also be used as a braising liquid for thighs and legs; just dilute it to the appropriate consistency with chicken stock or orange juice.

DARK CHOCOLATE & CHILE MOLE

Flavor Profile: *Bitter, Pungent*
Makes: *3 to 4 cups (705 to 940 ml)*

6 dried ancho chiles

2 tbsp (30 ml) extra-virgin olive oil, divided

1 tsp oregano

1½ tsp (3 g) allspice berries

½ tsp ground cumin seeds

½ tsp aniseed

½ tsp coriander seeds

2 tbsp (18 g) pumpkin seeds

1 yellow onion, diced

3–4 cloves garlic, chopped

1 (28-oz [794-g]) can tomato puree

2–3 dried prunes

1 cinnamon stick

1 slice stale bread, torn into chunks

2 oz (56 g) dark chocolate, minimum 80% cocoa, chopped

Salt, to taste

Grilled chicken, for serving

In a heavy pan over medium heat, toast the chiles in 1 tablespoon (15 ml) of olive oil until fragrant, about 5 minutes. Place a kettle of water on to boil. Place the chiles in a medium-sized bowl and add about ½ cup (120 ml) of the water just off the boil. Set it aside to cool for 10 minutes. When cool enough to handle, remove the stems and chop the chile peppers roughly.

While the chiles are cooling, wipe the pan clean with a paper towel and add the oregano, allspice, cumin seeds, aniseed, coriander seeds and pumpkin seeds. Toast just until fragrant, about 2 minutes. Transfer the spices to a spice grinder or use a mortar and pestle and grind them to a fine powder.

To the same pan, add the remaining tablespoon (15 ml) of olive oil, the onion and garlic. Cook until they're translucent, about 5 to 7 minutes. Add the toasted spices, tomato puree, chiles, prunes and cinnamon stick. Simmer over medium-low heat for about 30 minutes.

Remove the pan from the heat. Remove the cinnamon stick, stir in the bread and let it stand for 5 minutes. Using an immersion blender, puree the sauce until it's perfectly smooth. Stir in the dark chocolate. Season with salt to taste.

Serve over grilled chicken.

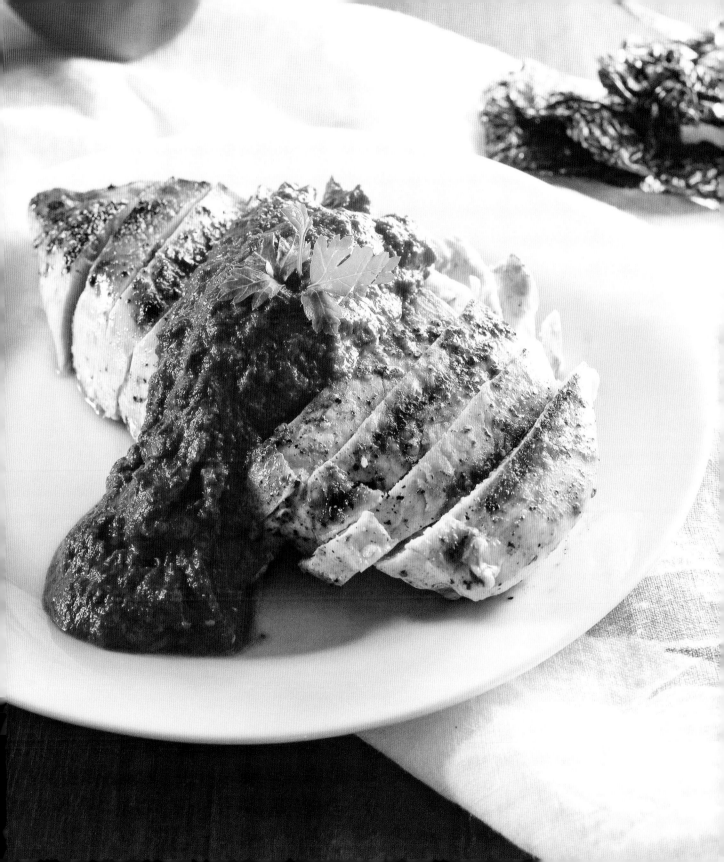

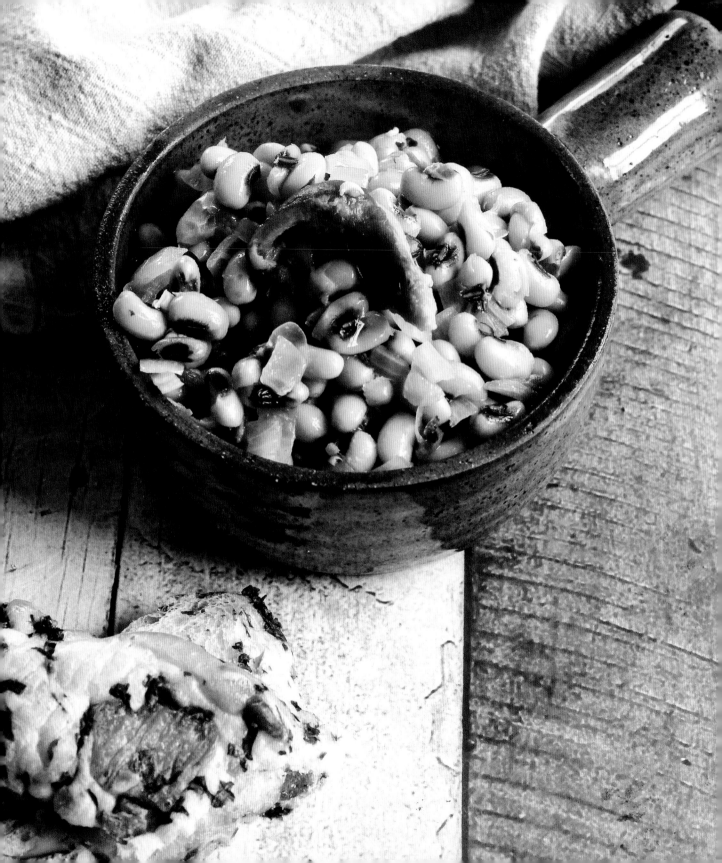

I've always been a fan of a warm bowl of bean soup, enriched with the smoky flavors of a ham hock. Navy or great northern beans have always been a pantry staple, but recently my attention has turned to clever little black-eyed peas.

A traditional New Year's food of the American South, black-eyed peas are thought to bring good luck—and they offer heart-friendly medicine. Fiber-rich black-eyed peas are associated with lowered blood pressure, reduced cholesterol and decreased insulin resistance. Bay leaves offer depth of flavor and counteract some of the gaseous effects of eating beans. This a meal that will positively stick to your ribs, and it is one that is good for you, too! Make this meal in your slow cooker for an easy, carefree dinner.

BLACK-EYED PEAS WITH HAM

Flavor Profile: *Sweet, Salty*

Serves: *4 to 6*

1 lb (450 g) dried black-eyed peas, soaked overnight and drained

1 large smoked ham hock

1 large onion, chopped

2–3 cloves garlic, minced

4 ribs celery, chopped

1 tsp smoked paprika, or to taste

1–2 bay leaves

Salt & freshly ground pepper, to taste

Add the black-eyed peas, ham hock, onion, garlic, celery, paprika and bay leaves to a large slow cooker. Set the pot to high and add enough water to cover all the ingredients by about 2 to 3 inches (5 to 7.5 cm). Cook, covered, for at least 8 to 10 hours, until the peas are perfectly tender and the meat on the ham hock falls away from the bones.

Remove the ham hock from the pot. Shred the remaining meat and add it back to the pot. Season with salt and pepper to taste.

Herbalist Tip
Soak your black-eyed peas for a minimum of 12 hours prior to preparing this meal to ensure tender beans. Do not salt the peas prior to cooking as this can toughen the skins.

Decadent desserts and heart health are strange bedfellows, but when polyphenol-laden chocolate and anthocyanin-rich hawthorn berries team up, all bets are off. A 2012 analysis of a 42 randomized, placebo-controlled and double-blind studies found substantial evidence that chocolate helped to reduce heart disease risk factors such as elevated triglycerides and high blood pressure, while also improving cholesterol ratios and decreasing insulin resistance. Marry heart-healthy chocolate with hawthorn berries, a traditional herbalist ally for cardiovascular function, and you have a dessert that really ticks all the boxes.

This flourless chocolate torte is created by first infusing the cream and butter with dried hawthorn berries. The berries impart a subtle berry flavor that provides nuance to the bold chocolate flavor. This torte is a perfectly celebratory dessert, and it is surprisingly easy to make.

CHOCOLATE & HAWTHORN BERRY FLOURLESS TORTE

Flavor Profile: *Bitter, Sweet, Sour*

Serves: *8, generously*

½ cup (112 g) unsalted butter, plus more for the pan

1 cup (100 g) dried hawthorn berries

⅔ cup (160 ml) heavy cream

⅔ cup (132 g) organic, unrefined sugar

Pinch of salt

8 eggs

12 oz (340 g) good-quality bittersweet chocolate pieces

Unsweetened cocoa, for dusting

Preheat your oven to 350°F (175°C, or gas mark 4).

Butter the bottom and sides of a 9-inch (23-cm) springform pan, lined with a round of parchment on the base. In a small saucepan, combine the hawthorn berries, butter and heavy cream. Bring them to a low simmer over low to medium heat. Reduce the heat and simmer very gently, stirring often, about 15 to 20 minutes, or until the cream mixture is slightly fragrant. Remove the pan from the heat and strain the mixture into a bowl through a fine-mesh sieve. Discard the spent berries.

In the bowl of a stand mixer with a whisk attachment, beat the sugar, salt and eggs on high speed until the mixture is very thick, pale and ribbon-y, about 5 to 8 minutes.

In a double boiler over gentle heat, combine the infused cream-butter mixture and the chocolate. Stir until it's melted and glossy. Temper the egg mixture by adding some of the chocolate. Fold the mixture together in thirds until evenly mixed. Take care not to overmix, deflating the volume.

Pour the mixture into the prepared springform pan. Bake for 35 to 40 minutes, until the top is somewhat dull and only the center jiggles somewhat when moved. It will NOT appear fully cooked when you remove it from the oven; it will set upon cooling. Do not overbake.

Allow the torte to cool for about 30 minutes before gently running a thin spatula or butter knife between the pan wall and torte. Carefully remove the outer ring. Continue to cool completely. Lightly dust the torte with unsweetened cocoa.

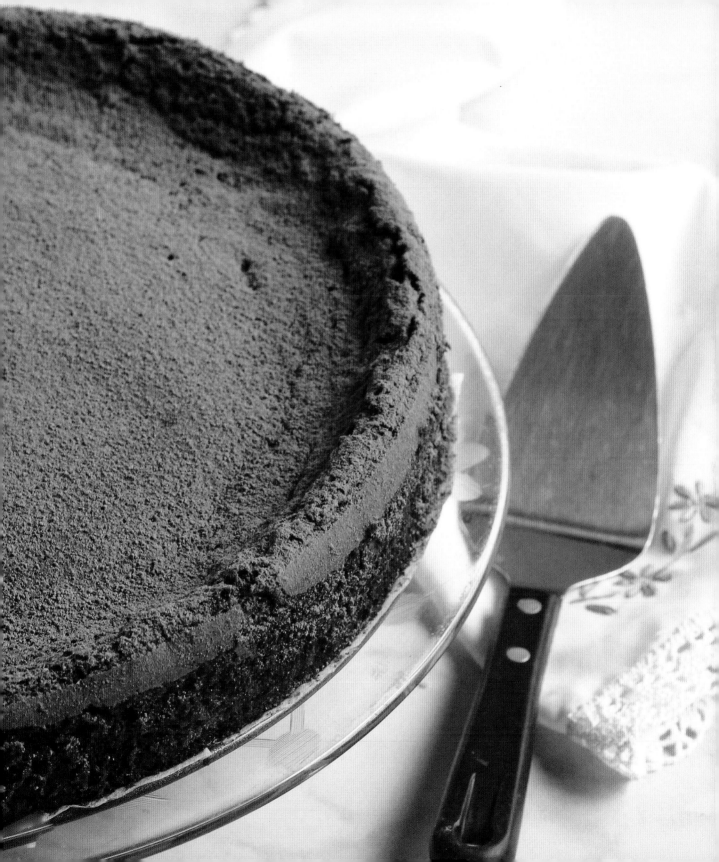

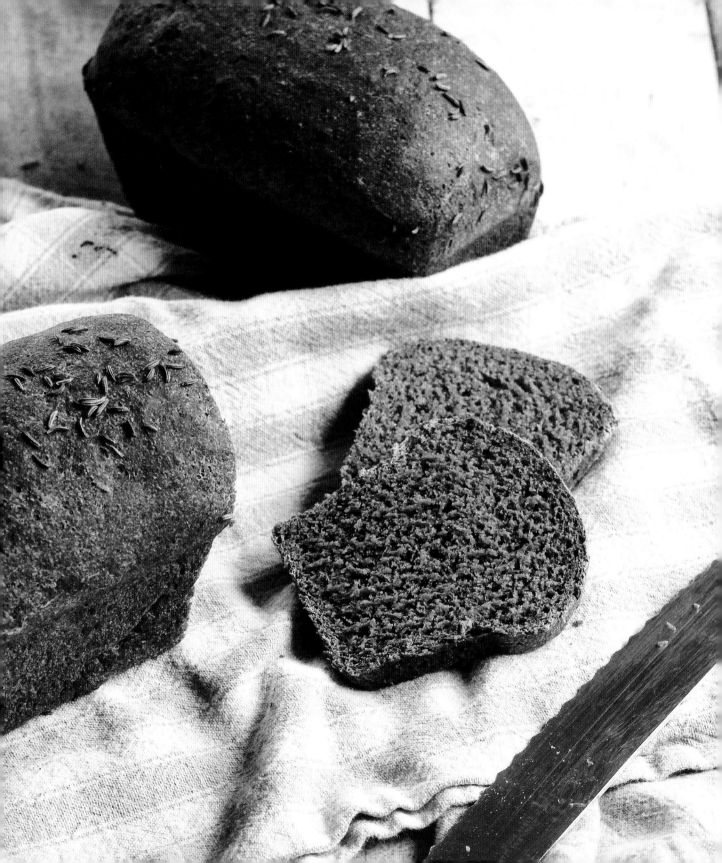

FIVE

RECIPES FOR A

HAPPY, HEALTHY BELLY

It is said that for some the path to the heart is through the stomach. I fall solidly into this camp. Designer clothes, florist deliveries, even jewels hold little appeal to me. But a marvelous meal prepared for me? I am putty in your hands. This girl loves food.

I am certainly not alone in my love of good food. But with food comes the matter of digestion. And let's face it, the modern mainstream diet isn't exactly geared toward a healthy gut. In fact, it is chock-full of sugars, fillers and otherwise undesirable, unappetizing and virtually indigestible substances. As a result, folks are falling victim to indigestion, leaky gut, heartburn and ulcers at an alarming rate.

I am of a firm belief that diet is the key to bringing our bellies back into a neutral, high-functioning state. And maintaining excellent digestion isn't difficult when we include a few of our flavors—namely bitter, sour, sweet and even pungent! The fresh anise-y notes of fennel are sure to sweeten a sour stomach. Caraway soothes gas and indigestion, and ginger gets to shine as the remedy for nausea.

Easy Refrigerator Dill Pickles (page 105) promote a hearty appetite, and they are the sure-fire cure for hiccups. Bitter, earthy Saffron Rock Candy (page 118) gets the digestive juices flowing. Fried Okra with Garlic Aioli (page 106) lends healing, soothing mucilage to the digestive tract. And pungent, warming Coconut Rice Pudding with Cardamom & Rose (page 113) is the perfect after-dinner treat to promote digestive action.

Gather all the goodness and give your belly a few delicious dishes to digest!

Everybody likes beans. Nobody likes the aftereffects. This soaking and slow-cooker method of preparing beans delivers a soft bean with intact flesh. The long soaking time also leaches the phytic acid, which is an "anti-nutrient" that interferes with digestion and nutrient absorption.

Earthy cumin promotes the secretion of bile to help break down fats for eased digestion. Lesser-known epazote is a traditional herb of the American Southwest and central America associated with decreased gas and bloating. Epazote can be found in some Latin American sections in the grocery store and specialty food shops, as well as online.

These beans are full of flavor. They are a meal in their own right served over rice and garnished with a few sprigs of fresh cilantro and crumbled cotija cheese.

PINTO BEANS WITH CUMIN & EPAZOTE

Flavor Profile: *Sweet, Pungent, Salty*
Serves: *6 to 8*

4 cups (770 g) dried pinto beans, sorted and rinsed

1 medium onion, chopped

2–3 cloves garlic, minced

1 tbsp (15 ml) extra-virgin olive oil

2 tbsp (14 g) ground cumin

2 tbsp (24 g) dried epazote leaves

1 tbsp (15 g) salt

For Serving

Cooked rice

Fresh cilantro

Crumbled cotija cheese

In a large bowl, cover the pinto beans with water. Soak them overnight or for at least 12 hours at room temperature.

The next day, drain and rinse the beans. In a medium-sized sauté pan over medium heat, sauté the onion and garlic in the olive oil until the onion is translucent, about 5 to 7 minutes.

Add the cumin and epazote and cook until fragrant, about 1 to 2 minutes. Add the beans, onion, garlic, spices and seasoning to your slow cooker. Add water to cover it. Cover with a lid and cook on the "low" setting for 10 to 12 hours.

After cooking, adjust the seasoning to your liking. Stir gently to avoid breaking up the beans. Spoon the beans over rice and serve with cilantro and cotija cheese.

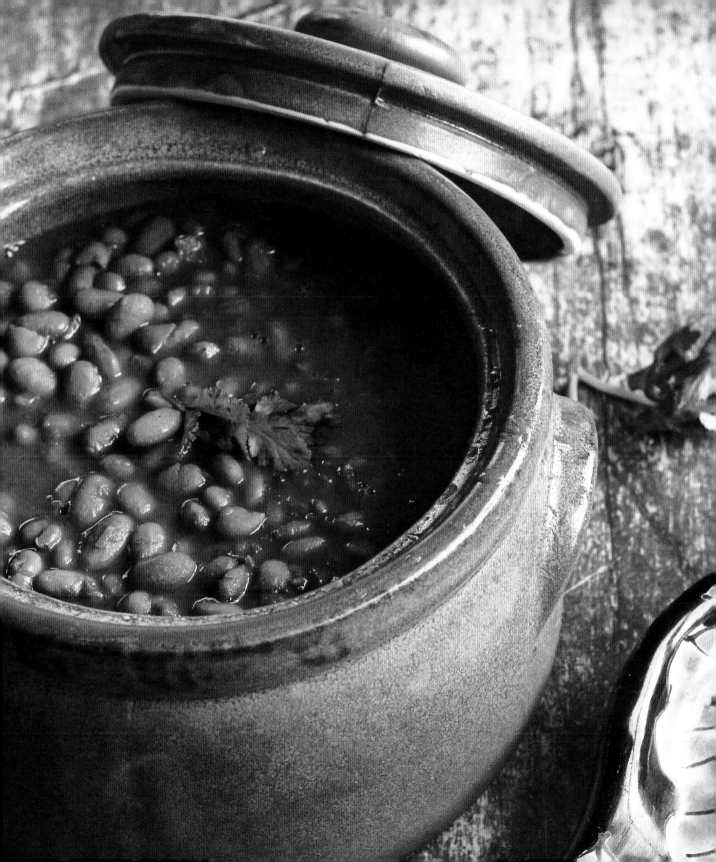

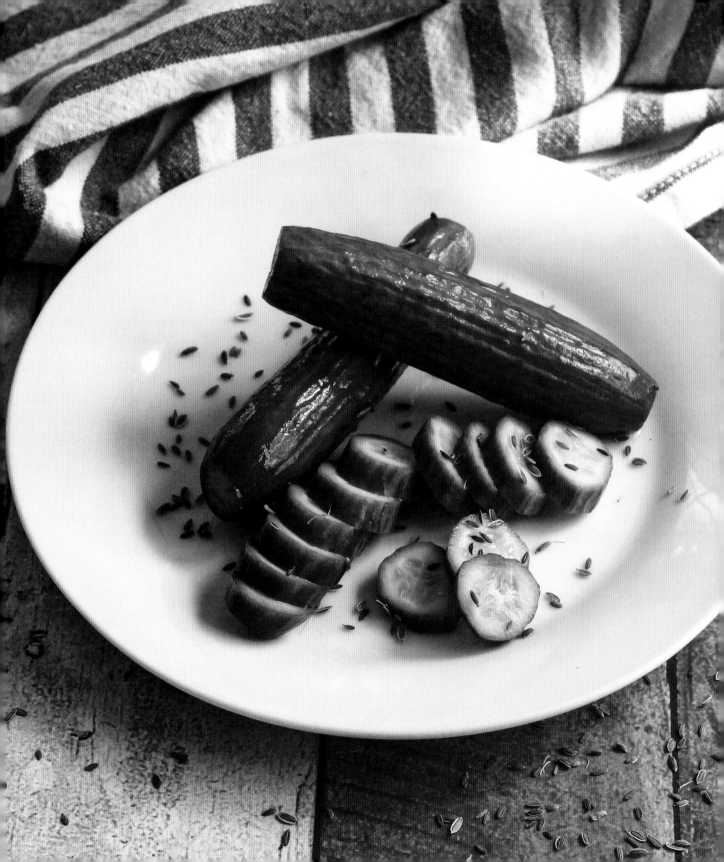

Dill is an unpraised hero of the culinary and medicinal herbal world. Viewed as the flavor of everybody's favorite pickle, it is so overlooked that we forget why dill works. Dill is an appetite stimulate, a sialagogue and antispasmodic. As such, dill stimulates the flow of digestive juices, promotes the production of saliva and relieves painful cramping and gas. Dill is also incredibly gentle and calming to an irritated stomach. This herb is even the silver bullet for painful, spasmodic hiccups. Don't believe me? Take a swig of the dill pickle brine the next time you have a bad case of the hiccups. You'll be rid of the nuisance immediately!

These refrigerator dills are a perfect snack or appetizer. The cucumbers can be prepared as spears, slices or even left whole. Brine time will vary due to the density of the cucumber.

EASY REFRIGERATOR DILL PICKLES

Flavor Profile: *Sour, Salty, Bitter, Pungent*

Makes: *2 quarts (1.9 L)*

4 cups (940 ml) water

2 cups (475 ml) white vinegar

2 tbsp (36 g) kosher salt

1 tsp sugar

10–12 pickling cucumbers (4–6 inches [10–15 cm]); 3–4 larger cucumbers (8–10 inches [20–25 cm]); OR 20–25 mini cucumbers (3–4 inches [7.5–10 cm])

6 large cloves garlic, peeled and smashed, divided

1 cup (9 g) fresh dill fronds, divided

2 tbsp (14 g) fresh dill seeds, divded

20 black peppercorns, divided

2 fresh grape leaves or green tea bags (optional)

In a small saucepan, heat the water, vinegar, salt and sugar until it's dissolved, about 2 to 3 minutes. Set it aside to cool for 30 minutes.

Slice or spear your cucumbers based on your personal preference. If you choose to keep your cucumbers whole, trim off the blossom ends.

Pack the cucumbers loosely into two sterilized quart-sized (940-ml) jars. Top each jar with 3 cloves of garlic, ½ cup (5 g) of dill fronds, 1 tablespoon (7 g) of dill seeds and 10 peppercorns per jar. If using grape leaves or tea bags, add one to each jar. Pour the cooled brine over the ingredients to cover them.

Screw on a tight-fitting lid. Brine them in the refrigerator for at least 1 week, then taste and judge the texture. Pickles should retain some crunch, but be somewhat translucent all the way through. Use them within 2 months.

Herbalist Tip
To maximize "crunch," adding a fresh grape leaf or a bag of green tea to the brining jar will reduce mushiness.

My husband used to live in the Midwest, and he also traveled quite a bit in the South as a youth and acquired a taste for okra. Being a solid Pacific Northwest girl myself, okra is just not a grocery or garden staple around here. Always curious about what draws folks to certain foods, I was particularly fascinated by my husband's fondness for okra. He is prone to poor gut health and ulcers due to a couple of factors in his childhood and adulthood. Okra is a member of the mallow family and contains healing, soothing mucilage that can have profound benefits for the digestive system. As such, okra is the perfect food for those plagued with stomach complaints of heat and burning.

When brainstorming recipes for this book, I considered gumbo or pickled okra, but settled on a somewhat naughty treat: fried okra. Because who doesn't want a naughty treat that isn't so naughty after all? I use frozen okra because that is what is regularly available; no need to thaw them before preparing this recipe. This simple coating browns to a nice golden hue while the okra cooks, resulting in a crunchy morsel without the slimy, mushy texture sometimes attributed to this vegetable. Dip it in garlic aioli for added yummy naughtiness.

FRIED OKRA WITH GARLIC AIOLI

Flavor Profile: *Sweet, Pungent*
Serves: *4*

⅓ cup (47 g) yellow cornmeal

⅓ cup plus 2 tbsp (58 g) all-purpose flour, divided

1 tsp paprika

½ tsp ground black pepper

½ tsp garlic powder

⅛ tsp cayenne pepper

2 cups (475 ml) sunflower or peanut oil, for frying

4 cups (225 g) chopped frozen okra

2 large eggs, beaten

Sea salt, to taste

Aioli

1 cup (225 g) homemade or store-bought mayonnaise

1 tbsp (15 ml) fresh lemon juice

3–4 cloves garlic, finely minced

Salt & freshly ground pepper, to taste

Combine the cornmeal, ⅓ cup (42 g) of flour, paprika, black pepper, garlic powder and cayenne pepper in a medium-sized bowl.

For the aioli, whisk together the mayonnaise, lemon juice and garlic, then season it with salt and pepper to taste. Set the aioli aside.

Preheat a medium-sized saucepan filled with the oil over medium-high heat. Toss the frozen okra with 2 tablespoons (16 g) of flour, then dip them into the egg before dredging them in the cornmeal mixture.

Check the oil by placing one piece of coated okra into it. It should sizzle and bubbles should form immediately. Fry the okra in small batches for 3 to 5 minutes until deeply golden. Lift with a slotted spoon and drain them on a paper towel. When done frying, toss the okra with sea salt to taste. Serve with the aioli for dipping.

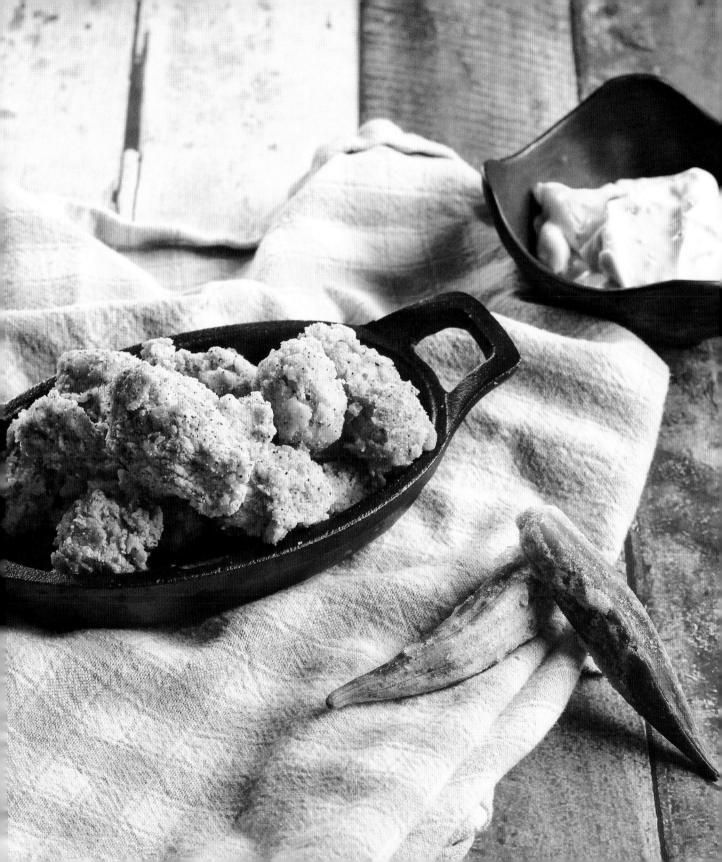

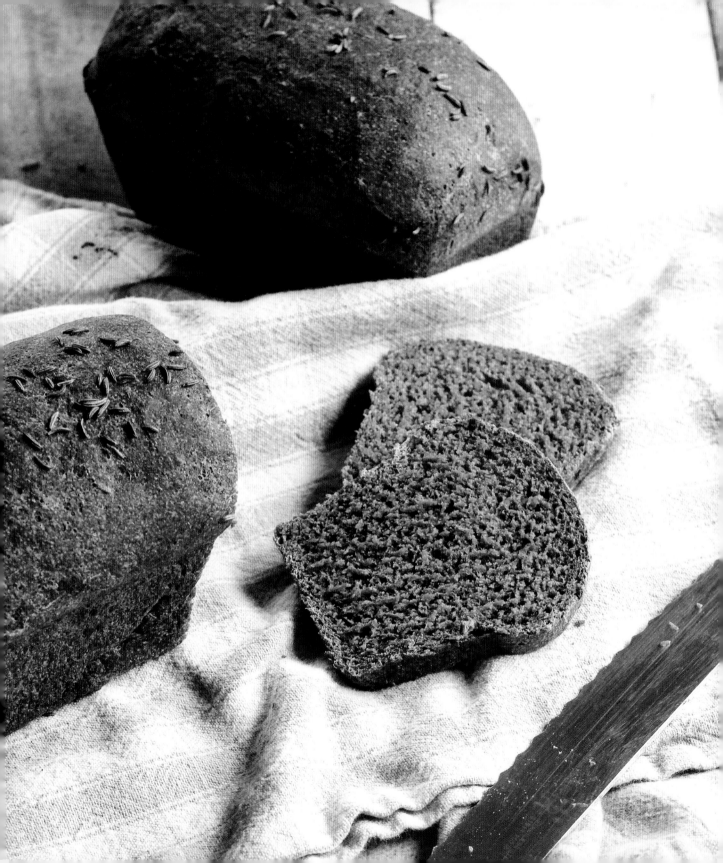

I have the fondest memories of eating mini sandwiches on Christmas day. Savory cured meats and creamy cheeses piled on a dark dense bread—and the unmistakable flavor of caraway that lingered on my palate.

When I settled on the concept for this book, I knew that I had to re-create this flavor from my childhood. I reached out to my dear friend and sourdough expert Courtney Queen of ButterforAll.com for a little fermentation guidance. So, with Courtney's help, I have now realized the nostalgic flavors of those bygone Christmas days and ended up with a belly-friendly bread. The slow fermentation of these rye loaves makes for highly digestible bread, while the caraway seeds promote good digestion and eliminate gas and bloating.

RYE & CARAWAY MINI LOAVES

Flavor Profile: *Sweet, Pungent, Sour*
Makes: *2 mini loaves*

2½ cups (320 g) rye flour

1 cup (140 g) bread flour

½ cup (125 g) active sourdough starter at 100% hydration

¼ cup (60 ml) molasses

2 tbsp (12 g) caraway seeds, plus 1 tbsp (6 g) for topping bread

1¾ tsp (10 g) sea salt

1 cup (235 ml) unchlorinated water

Herbalist Tip
You can create a simple sourdough starter using one-part organic all-purpose flour to one-part unchlorinated water. Ferment it at room temperature. Remove half the volume each day, replacing it with an equal volume of water and flour. Do this for 10 to 14 days until the starter develops a characteristic sour aroma. Feeding the starter every day will ensure it remains in an "active" fermentation state. You can store the starter in the refrigerator if it is not being fed at least every other day. To reactivate the starter, take it out of the fridge and feed it once or twice a day for 2 to 3 days.

The night before baking, mix the flours, sourdough starter, molasses, caraway, salt and water into a dough. Knead the dough on a lightly floured surface until smooth. Loosely shape the dough into a ball, place it in a clean bowl, cover and proof it overnight at room temperature, about 8 to 10 hours.

The next morning, punch the dough down in the bowl and turn it out on a floured surface. Loosely shape the dough into a ball. Cut the dough into two equal portions. Let the dough rest for 5 minutes.

Shape each half into a mini loaf by patting the dough into a rectangle. Fold and press the top toward the center, and then fold and press the bottom toward the center. Turn the loaf over and let it rest seam-side down, about 5 to 10 minutes.

Brush the top of each loaf with water and sprinkle them with caraway seeds. Transfer the mini loaves to greased mini bread pans, about 5½ x 3 inches (14 x 7.5 cm), to continue fermenting. Let the dough proof in the pans at room temperature to double in size, about 1 to 2 hours.

Preheat your oven to 400°F (200°C, or gas mark 6). Bake in the oven for 30 minutes.

Remove the loaves from the oven and let them rest in the pans for 10 minutes. Remove the loaves to wire racks to cool completely before slicing.

If you have had the pleasure of drinking a chai tea latte, then this crème brûlée will be a special treat. Chai is a traditional Indian drink that is cherished for its stomach-calming nature. Here, ginger and cardamom encourage digestion, and true cinnamon even discourages spikes in blood glucose, making this a dessert with a myriad of health benefits.

Crème brûlée is not difficult to make, but it takes some time and attention. The result is a silky-smooth custard with exotic chai flavors, topped with a glaze of brûléed sugar. Despite being a dairy-rich dessert, the inclusion of chai spices makes this crème brûlée decidedly less heavy, but altogether heavenly. The dry spice blend is perfect for teas and lattes, as well as infusing into the custard for this sumptuous dessert.

CHAI-SPICED CRÈME BRÛLÉE

Flavor Profile: *Pungent, Sweet*
Serves: *4 to 6*

Chai Spice Blend

1 cup (175 g) cinnamon chips

¼ cup (14 g) cardamom pods, crushed

¼ cup (14 g) star anise, crushed

2 tbsp (14 g) dried ginger granules

2 tbsp (12 g) fennel seeds

1 tsp coarsely ground black pepper, or more depending on your taste

Custard

¾ cup (175 ml) whole milk

¾ cup (175 ml) heavy cream

3 tbsp (30 g) chai spice blend

5 large egg yolks

¼ cup (85 g) honey or sugar

Pinch of kosher salt

Topping

2 tsp (9 g) sugar per ramekin

To make the chai spice blend, combine the cinnamon chips, cardamom, star anise, ginger granules, fennel seeds and pepper in a jar with a tight-fitting lid. Cover with the lid and shake well to combine.

To make the custard, start by preheating your oven to 325°F (170°C, or gas mark 3).

In a small saucepan over medium heat, add the whole milk, heavy cream and chai spice. Bring to a gentle simmer, about 5 to 7 minutes, stirring gently so as to not incorporate air into the mixture. Remove the pan from the heat and set it aside.

In a medium-sized bowl, whisk together the egg yolks, honey and salt until they're well combined, about 15 to 20 seconds. Using a ladle, add a small amount of the infused milk and cream to the egg-and-honey mixture, stirring well to combine them, then add the rest of the milk mixture slowly while continuing to stir.

Strain the custard through a fine-mesh sieve and pour it into individual 5-ounce (148-ml) ramekins, leaving about ¼ to ½ inch (6 mm to 1.3 cm) headspace. This recipe will fill 4 to 6 ramekins depending on the fill height and the size of the eggs used. Place the ramekins in a deep, rimmed baking dish and fill the dish with hot water about halfway up the sides of the ramekins. Tent the dish loosely with foil. Cook in the oven for 40 to 45 minutes until the outer half of the custard is set but the center still wobbles slightly.

Remove the baking dish from the oven. Cool and chill the custard in the refrigerator for at least 4 to 6 hours or overnight. To serve, sprinkle the tops of each custard evenly with 2 teaspoons (9 g) of sugar. Using a small blowtorch, blaze the sugar until it's amber and well caramelized. If you do not have a torch, you can use the broiler of the oven; watch closely so they don't burn. Serve immediately.

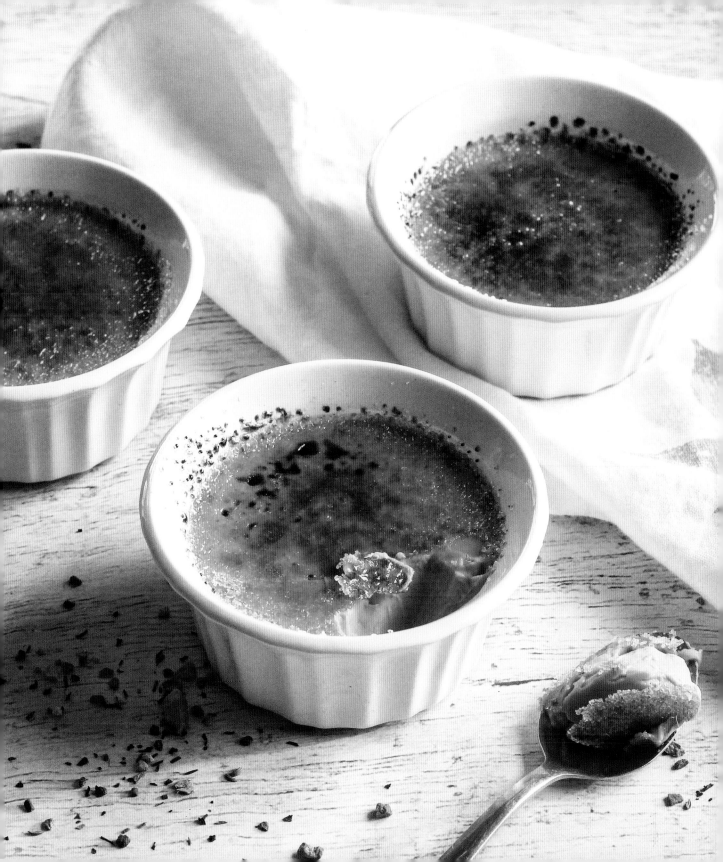

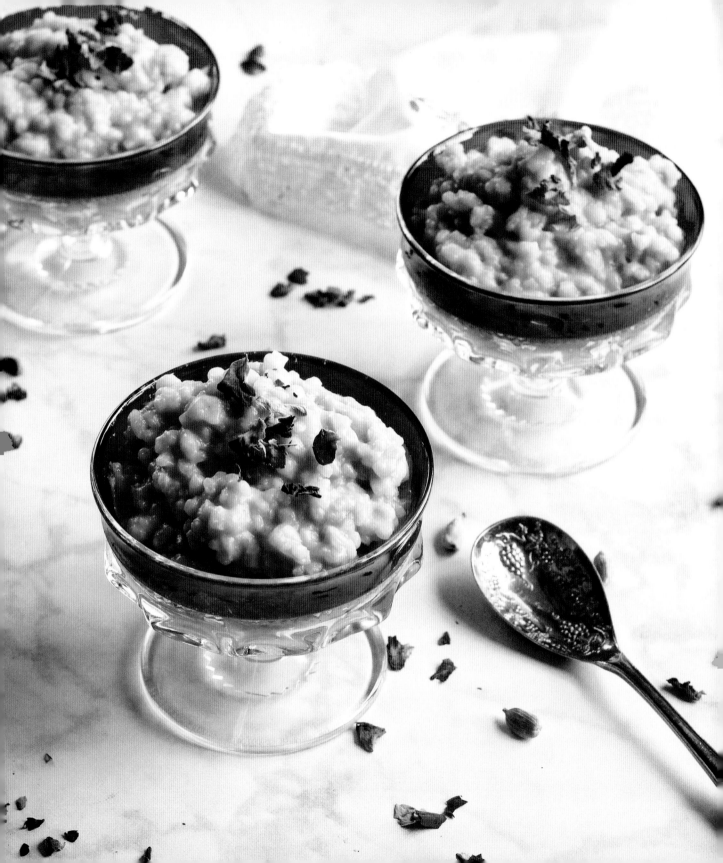

Creamy and exotic. That is the best pair of descriptors for this unctuous dessert. Rice pudding is a delicious comfort food, full of sugar and dairy. I lightened the dish by replacing traditional dairy with coconut milk, and I elevated it to something really special with cardamom and rose.

Cardamom is a great stimulator of digestive action and is incredibly soothing to a sour stomach. Rose is a gentle astringent, helping to firm lax digestive tissues and arrest mucus-y discharges that can irritate the stomach and bowel. Use short-grain arborio rice for this pudding to impart the ultimate silky, creamy custard-like texture.

COCONUT RICE PUDDING WITH CARDAMOM & ROSE

Flavor Profile: *Pungent, Sweet, Salty*

Serves: *4 to 6*

1½ cups (355 ml) water

¾ cup (150 g) uncooked short-grain white rice (such as arborio)

1 egg

2 cups (475 ml) full-fat unsweetened coconut milk, divided

2 tbsp (about 2 g) dried rose petals, plus more for garnish

1 tbsp (4 g) lightly crushed green cardamom pods (about 7–8)

⅓ cup (115 g) honey or sugar

¼ tsp salt

In a medium-sized saucepan, bring the water to a boil over high heat. Stir in the rice, reduce the heat to low and cover the pan. Cook for 20 minutes, stirring occasionally to release the starch from the rice grains. After cooking, remove the rice from the heat and set it aside.

Meanwhile, whisk together the egg and ½ cup (120 ml) of coconut milk. Set it aside.

In a medium-sized saucepan, add the remaining coconut milk, rose petals, cardamom, honey and salt. Bring it to a simmer over medium heat. Continue to cook for about 5 to 7 minutes, until the coconut is fragrant. Remove the pan from the heat and strain it through a fine-mesh sieve. Return the infused milk to the saucepan and add the cooked rice. Cook over medium-low heat for 15 to 20 minutes, stirring frequently, until the mixture is creamy and thickened. Remove about 1 tablespoon (13 g) of the rice mixture and whisk it into the coconut milk–egg mixture to temper it. Add the tempered mixture to the rice mixture and stir it well to combine them. Remove from the heat.

This pudding can be served warm or chilled.

These little digestive biscuits are big on flavor and texture. Rich, golden cornmeal offers these biscuits a light, airy texture, while anise-y fennel seeds do all the digestive heavy lifting. Fennel stimulates the appetite, encourages digestion and alleviates sensations of gas and bloating.

These digestive biscuits are ever-so-slightly sweet, making them perfect for an after-dinner snack. They are even more wonderful with a cheese and charcuterie board. These biscuits are so delicious that you might find yourself eating more than a handful!

CORNMEAL & FENNEL SEED DIGESTIVE BISCUITS

Flavor Profile: *Sweet, Salty*
Makes: *24 to 30 cookies*

1 cup (125 g) all-purpose flour
1 cup (125 g) yellow cornmeal
1 tsp baking powder
½ cup (100 g) sugar
1 tsp sea salt
2 tsp (4 g) fennel seeds
8 tbsp (112 g) butter, cubed and softened to room temperature
¾ cup (175 ml) whole milk

In the bowl of a food processor, pulse the flour, cornmeal, baking powder, sugar, salt and fennel seeds until they're well mixed. In short bursts, pulse the butter into the flour mixture until it resembles a coarse meal. Add the milk and pulse again until a cohesive dough forms.

Turn the dough out onto a well-floured surface. Without overworking the dough, form two dough balls and flatten each into a small disc. Wrap them in plastic film and chill them in the refrigerator for at least 30 minutes.

Meanwhile, preheat your oven to 350°F (175°C, or gas mark 4) and line cookie sheets with parchment paper. Roll out the dough on a well-floured surface until it measures about ⅛ inch (3 mm) thick. Using a pizza wheel or a rotary dough crimping tool, cut individual cookies in roughly 1 x 2–inch (2.5 x 5–cm) rectangles. Transfer them carefully to the lined baking sheet. Pierce each one once with the tines of a fork to prevent puffing in the oven.

Bake for 18 to 20 minutes, or until they're lightly golden, rotating the sheet about halfway through the baking time to ensure even browning. Cool them for at least 10 minutes on the baking sheet, then transfer them to a wire rack to continue cooling. Do not underbake. These biscuits are best cooked until firm for a cracker-like snap.

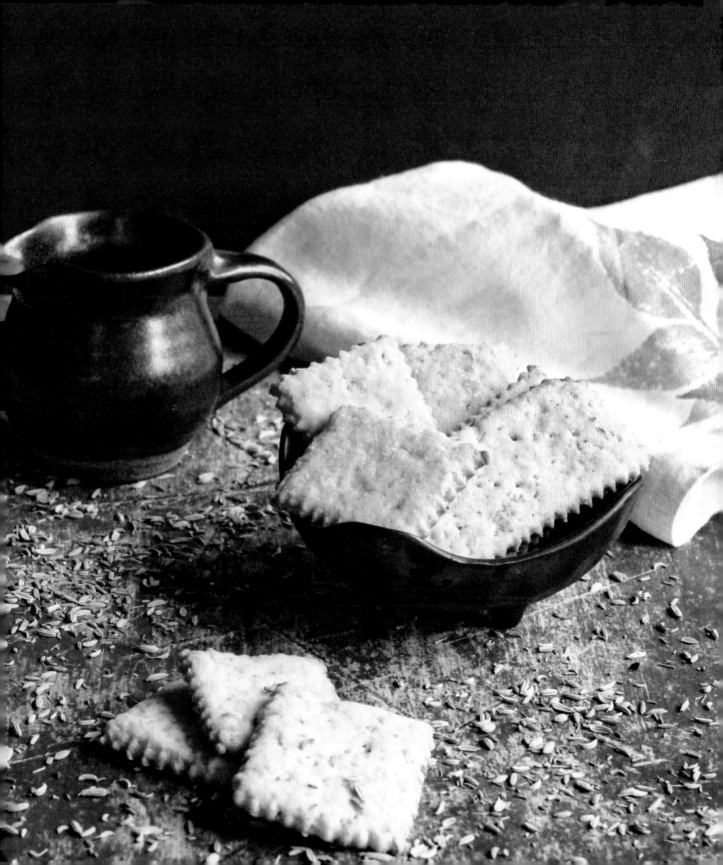

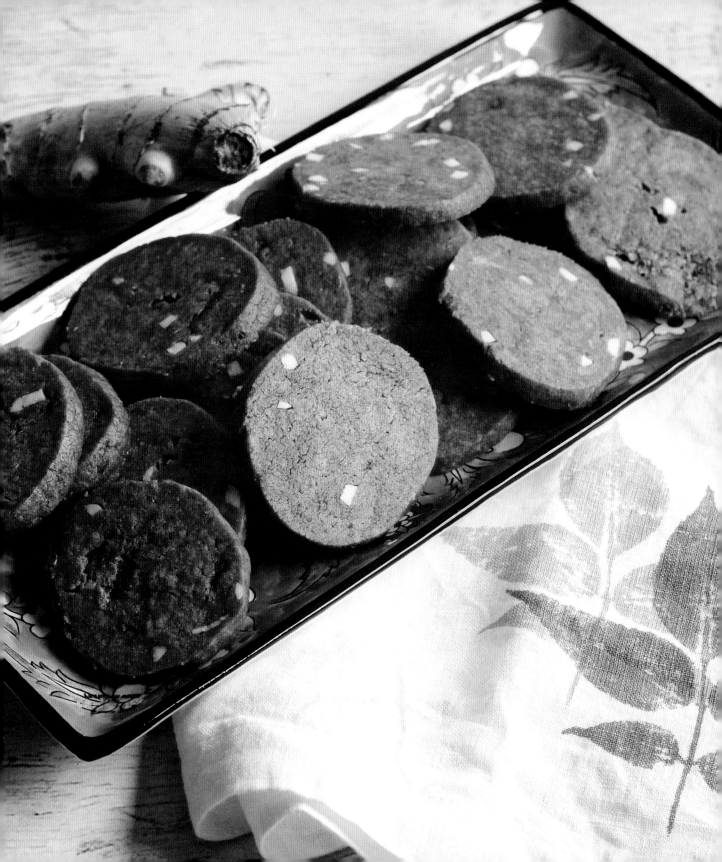

Ginger is, without a doubt, one of my favorites in the culinary and medicinal toolbox. Warm, spicy and pungent, ginger offers a great deal of flavor while also easing digestive upset and cramping.

These ginger thins are prefect for long road trips, for those prone to motion sickness, and perhaps they could even quell a bout of seasickness. They are ideal for the expectant mother to stave off morning sickness and a great soother of nausea, vomiting and even menstrual cramping.

These cookies are simple and tasty, and they bring great immediate relief to those who take a nibble! They are also absolutely delicious crumbled over the Dairy-Free Tropical Fruit "Nice Cream" with Ginger (page 122).

SOOTHING GINGER THINS

Flavor Profile: *Pungent, Sweet*

Makes: *24 to 30 cookies*

6 tbsp (83 g) butter, softened

½ cup plus 2 tbsp (125 g) sugar, divided

3 tbsp (45 ml) molasses

1¼ cups (157 g) all-purpose flour

½ tsp baking soda

1 tsp ground ginger

¼ tsp ground cloves

⅛ tsp salt

¼ cup (26 g) sliced almonds (optional)

In a stand mixer or with an electric beater, cream together the softened butter and ½ cup (100 g) of sugar. Scrape the sides of the bowl and add the molasses, then beat again until it's fluffy and well combined, about 30 to 40 seconds.

In a separate bowl, sift together the flour, baking soda, ginger, cloves and salt. Add the flour mixture to the butter mixture and mix together by hand until it's well combined. Stir in the almonds, if using. The dough will be quite soft.

Spoon the dough onto plastic film or waxed paper. Form a log about 7 inches (18 cm) long, 1½ inches (3.5 cm) wide and 1 inch (2.5 cm) deep. No need to be super precise. Freeze this dough for at least 8 hours or overnight.

Preheat your oven to 350°F (175°C, or gas mark 4).

Line a baking sheet with parchment paper or a silicone mat. While the dough is still frozen, unwrap it and slice it into rounds about ⅛ inch (3 mm) thick. Place the slices on the lined baking sheet, sprinkle the tops with the remaining 2 tablespoons (25 g) sugar and bake for about 8 to 10 minutes. Remove them from the oven and allow the cookies to cool completely on the sheet tray before removing them. Store them in an airtight container for up to 1 week.

Herbalist Tip

Give yourself plenty of time to prepare as this dough MUST freeze overnight for a perfectly crunchy cookie!

I have enjoyed cooking with saffron on rare occasions when I am feeling indulgent—and flush with cash. But it was only a few years ago that I became aware of the therapeutic value of this precious spice. Chitchatting with a friend and neighbor about herbal medicine one morning, she mentioned that her favorite childhood remedy for an upset stomach was the saffron rock candy that her Persian father always offered. My friend dipped into her pantry and produced a small cellophane bag of the crystallized candy. "Here, try some," she said. I did and I immediately knew that this was a recipe I needed to try out.

Saffron aids in digestion and quells the feeling of stomach upset and nausea. This recipe is equal parts mad scientist and Willy Wonka—making for a fun project for little ones to observe. While I would hardly suggest rock candy as an everyday recipe, this might just make a perfect treat for after a rich meal!

SAFFRON ROCK CANDY

Flavor Profile: *Bitter, Sweet*

Makes: *16 candy pops*

2 wide-mouth pint-size (475-ml) jars

12 wooden skewers (8 of them cut in half and pointy ends removed)

2 cups (475 ml) water

Pinch of saffron

4 cups (800 g) sugar

Sterilize the jars with boiling water. Tape 4 cut skewers perpendicular to one long skewer so that the skewers hang about 1 inch (2.5 cm) from the bottom of the jar when the longer skewer is suspended on the rim.

In a medium-sized saucepan, add the water and saffron. Bring it to a boil over medium-high heat. Add the sugar 1 cup (200 g) at a time, stirring until all the sugar is dissolved, before adding the next cup. When all the sugar is dissolved, remove the pan from the heat and cool for 10 minutes.

Carefully suspend two skewers set up from the top of both jars, allowing about ¾ inch (2 cm) between the horizontal skewers and ensuring the suspended skewers are not too close to the sides of the jar. Pour the sugar solution into the jars, leaving adequate headspace to avoid spilling.

Cover them with plastic film and set the jars in a cool, dark place. Crystals will start to form on the skewers within about 4 hours and will continue to build as long as there is liquid sugar solution in the jar.

Check daily, and in about 7 days you should start seeing crystals form. Depending on temperature and humidity, your candies should be well formed in 10 to 20 days. When happy with the rock candies, remove the candy sticks from the solution and dry them on a wire rack, wrap them in cellophane or store them in an airtight container.

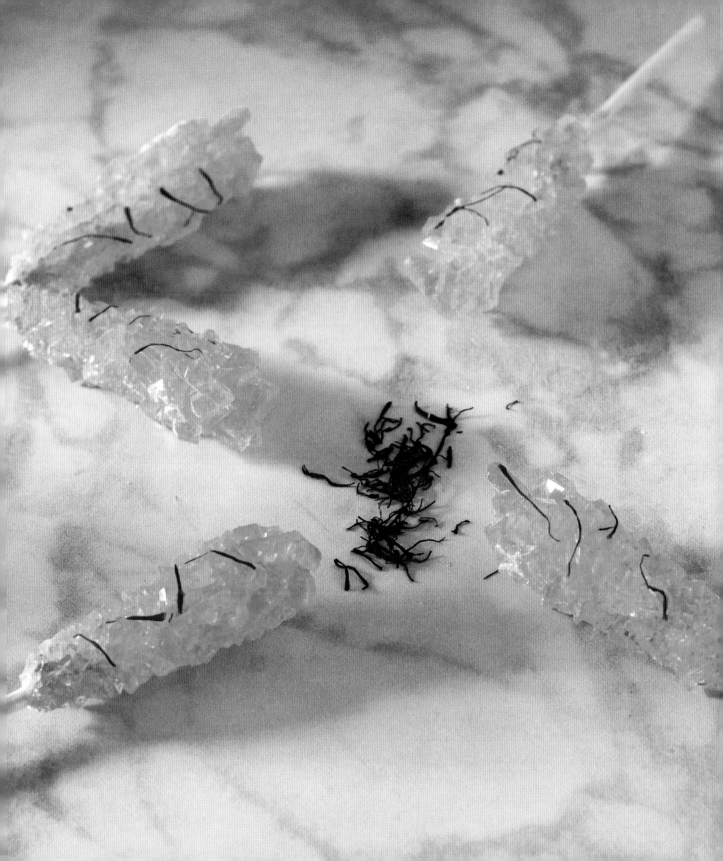

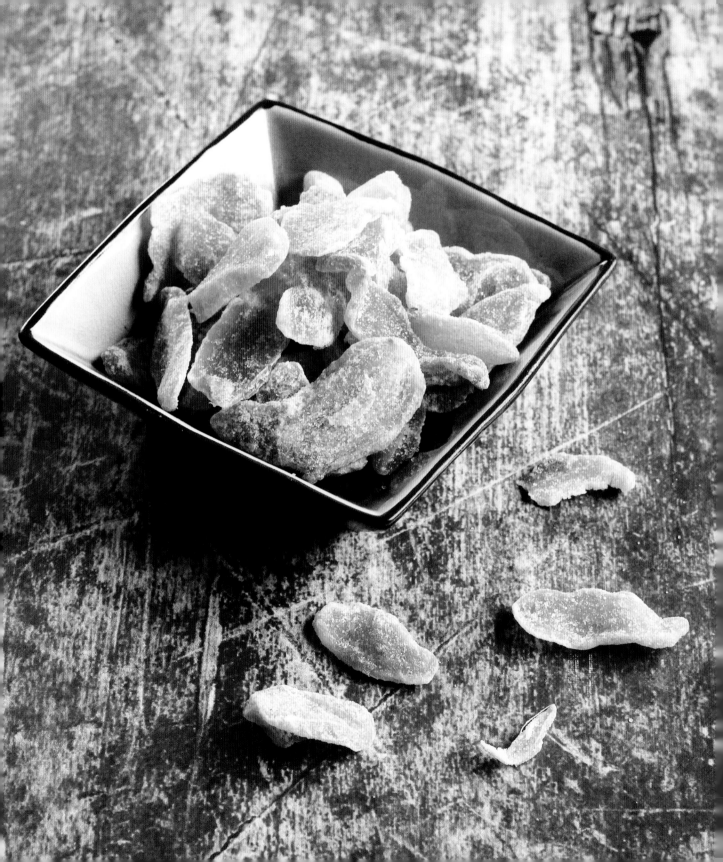

Ginger is a favored herb, known to herbalists, chefs and regular folks alike. The pungent, spicy rhizome quells nausea and upset stomach caused by pregnancy and motion sickness. Additionally, it relieves the sensation of gas and bloating, making it a favored ingredient in cooking.

These crystallized ginger candies are downright festive in their glittering glory. They are easy to make and store well, so keep a supply of these spicy lifesavers on hand!

CRYSTALLIZED GINGER CANDIES

Flavor Profile: *Pungent, Sweet*
Makes: *About 2 cups (450 g)*

½ lb (226 g) fresh ginger root
1 cup (200 g) sugar, plus more for coating

Peel the ginger root. Using a mandolin or a knife, cut the root into ⅛-inch (3-mm) slices for a crunchier candy, or up to ¼ inch (6 mm) for a chewier result.

Add the ginger slices to a small saucepan and cover them with water. Bring it to a boil, then reduce the heat to medium-low, cover and simmer for about 30 minutes.

After 30 minutes, strain the ginger through a fine-mesh sieve into a small bowl, reserving ¼ cup (60 ml) of the ginger liquid. Return the ginger slices and reserved liquid back to the saucepan. Add the sugar.

Bring the mixture to a boil over medium-high heat. Boil until the mixture reads 225°F (107°C) on a candy thermometer. This is referred to as the thread stage in candy-making; a spoon dipped in the syrup should result in long, thin threads dripping from the spoon.

Remove the pan from the heat. Pour the mixture through a fine-mesh sieve; reserve the resulting syrup for other uses, such as mixing with sparkling water or club soda for a makeshift ginger ale. Place the ginger slices on a wire rack in a single layer and dry them for 18 to 24 hours.

When the ginger is mostly dry, but still slightly sticky, toss them in a bowl of granulated sugar to coat. Place the ginger candies in a serving bowl and keep them dry, or store them in a container with an airtight lid.

Herbalist Tip
I like to pick organic ginger with few "knobs" so that I can maximize the size of the resulting candy.

Here is a guilt-free dessert that tastes amazing and can even atone for a multitude of dietary sins. Tropical fruits such as papaya and pineapple contain enzymes that promote vigorous and healthy digestion, preventing the feelings of bloating after a robust meal. Mango and strawberries add fiber and regulate proper bowel function. Coconut milk contributes a creamy texture and subtle tropical flavor. The addition of Crystallized Ginger Candies (page 121) stimulates peristalsis—the wave-like motions of the stomach wall necessary for good digestion— and reduces nausea caused by over-indulgence.

Dairy-free and containing no added sugar, this naturally sweet dessert is delightfully fruity on its own. It is over-the-top delicious with a few crumbled Soothing Ginger Thins (page 117).

DAIRY-FREE TROPICAL FRUIT "NICE CREAM" WITH GINGER

Flavor Profile: *Sour, Sweet*

Serves: *4 to 6*

½ cup (122 g) frozen pineapple chunks

½ cup (90 g) frozen papaya chunks

½ cup (85 g) frozen mango chunks

½ cup (100 g) frozen sliced strawberries

½ cup (120 ml) orange juice or tropical fruit juice blend (100% juice)

1 (13.5-oz [398-ml]) can full-fat unsweetened coconut milk

2 tbsp (30 g) minced Crystallized Ginger Candies (page 121)

Place the frozen fruit and juice into a food processor or blender. Process them until the fruit is well chopped but still slightly chunky, about 30 seconds. Add the coconut milk and process this until the mixture is well incorporated. Fold in the crystallized ginger by hand.

Serve immediately in well-chilled bowls or churn in an ice cream maker according to the appliance directions for better scoop-ability and better storage in the freezer.

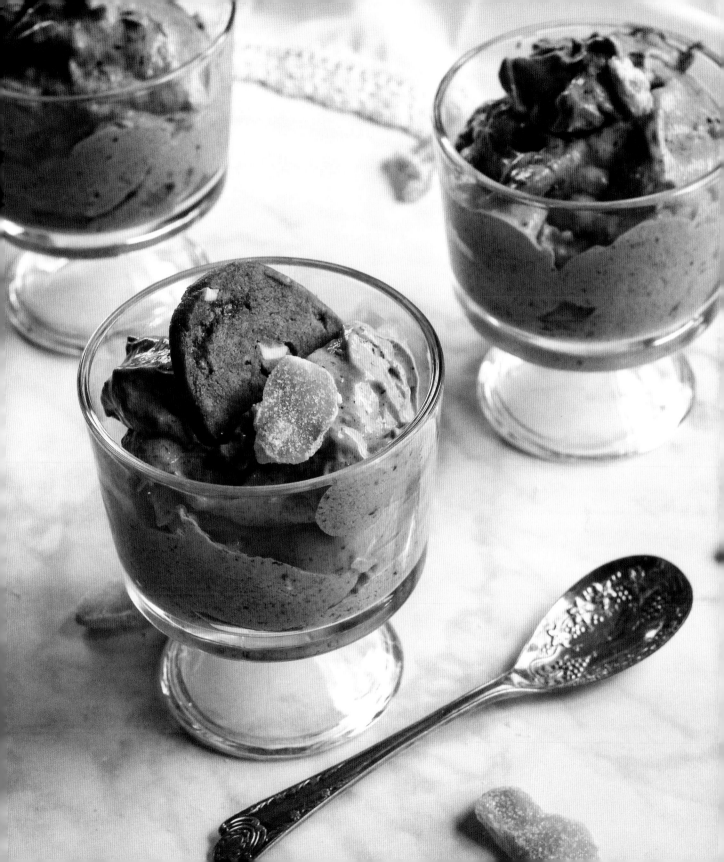

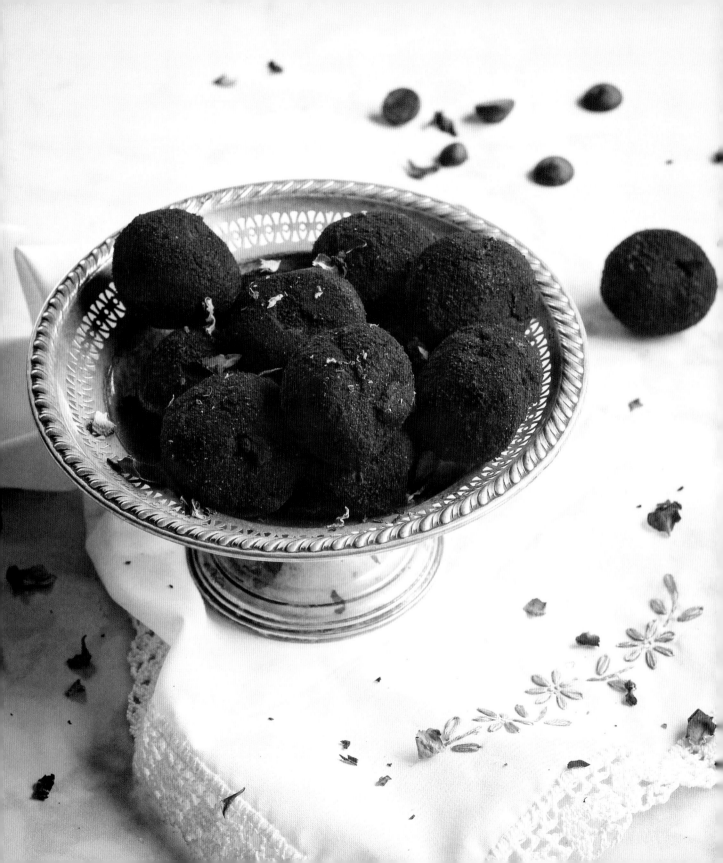

SIX

RECIPES TO

REV UP YOUR REPRODUCTIVE SYSTEM

Did I set out to write a chapter of recipes intended to make you blush? Maybe. But more importantly, I didn't want to gloss over a subject that I feel goes under-discussed. Reproductive and sexual health are pretty important factors in the survival of the human race, and a disordered reproductive system can have a serious impact outside of sexual and reproductive health. So quit blushing already.

We can take charge of our reproductive health—and much of that can be done without pharmaceutical intervention. Diet plays a key role in supporting sexual and reproductive health, from helping us to maintain a healthy body weight to contributing the essential building blocks needed to support hormonal health.

Reproductive health isn't as clear-cut flavor-wise as other bodily systems are. Savory herbs—such as parsley, tarragon and sage—cool and detoxify. Warming spices—such as cinnamon and ginger—arouse and awaken. Try sweet Silky-Smooth Hummus with Homemade Tahini (page 126) to help regulate blood glucose and, in turn, support hormonal health in both men and women. The Zingy Grapefruit & Rose Hip Curd (page 138) and the Goji Berry & Strawberry Smoothie (page 142) protect cells vital in the production of reproductive hormones. And because I maybe wanted you to blush just a little bit, I have included a couple of aphrodisiac recipes. Oysters on the Half Shell with Mignonette Sauce (page 133) or Rose & Maca Hand-Rolled Truffles (page 134), anyone?

Never forget that you are in charge of your reproductive health—and find the foods that put you in all the good moods!

The secret to a tasty, creamy hummus is a good tahini. Tahini is a paste made from ground sesame seeds, and it is incredibly easy to make from scratch. Sesame seeds themselves support fertility and reproductive health by promoting progesterone production. Balanced progesterone levels help to maintain fertility and regular menses, as well as decrease moodiness and headaches. Combined with the high fiber content of the garbanzo beans, this hummus is a great, healthy snack. Garbanzo beans (chickpeas) also offer fiber essential to regulating blood glucose—which, in turn, aids in hormonal balance. Cumin has been indicated to help fight age-related bone loss.

SILKY-SMOOTH HUMMUS WITH HOMEMADE TAHINI

Flavor Profile: *Sweet, Pungent*

Makes: *About 2 cups (500 g)*

Tahini

1 cup (140 g) sesame seeds, toasted

2–4 tbsp (30–60 ml) sesame oil

Salt, to taste

Hummus

1 (15-oz [425-g]) can garbanzo beans, drained

½ tsp baking soda

¼ cup (60 ml) fresh lemon juice

2–3 cloves garlic, minced

½ tsp fine sea salt, or to taste

½ tsp ground cumin

2–4 tbsp (30–60 ml) ice water, plus more as needed

1 tbsp (15 ml) extra-virgin olive oil, plus more for garnish

For Serving

Fresh vegetables

Grilled flatbread

To make the tahini, in a food processor, grind the sesame seeds into a fine meal. With the processor running, slowly drizzle in the sesame oil and puree until the mixture is perfectly smooth. Add a pinch or two of salt to taste. Set aside ½ cup (125 g) to use in this recipe.

For the hummus, in a small saucepan, cover the garbanzo beans with water. Add the baking soda and bring it to a gentle simmer over medium heat. Cook for 20 minutes and then drain the beans. Allow them to cool for at least 20 minutes.

In a food processor, add the lemon juice, garlic, salt, cumin and cooled garbanzo beans. Puree well. Add the reserved tahini and the ice water. Puree until it's silky-smooth and fluffy, then, with the food processor running, drizzle in the olive oil.

Spoon the hummus into a serving bowl and drizzle it with more olive oil. Serve with vegetables and flatbread.

Herbalist Tip

Focus on eating this hummus during the luteal phase (the latter 2 weeks) of your cycle to increase your progesterone level naturally.

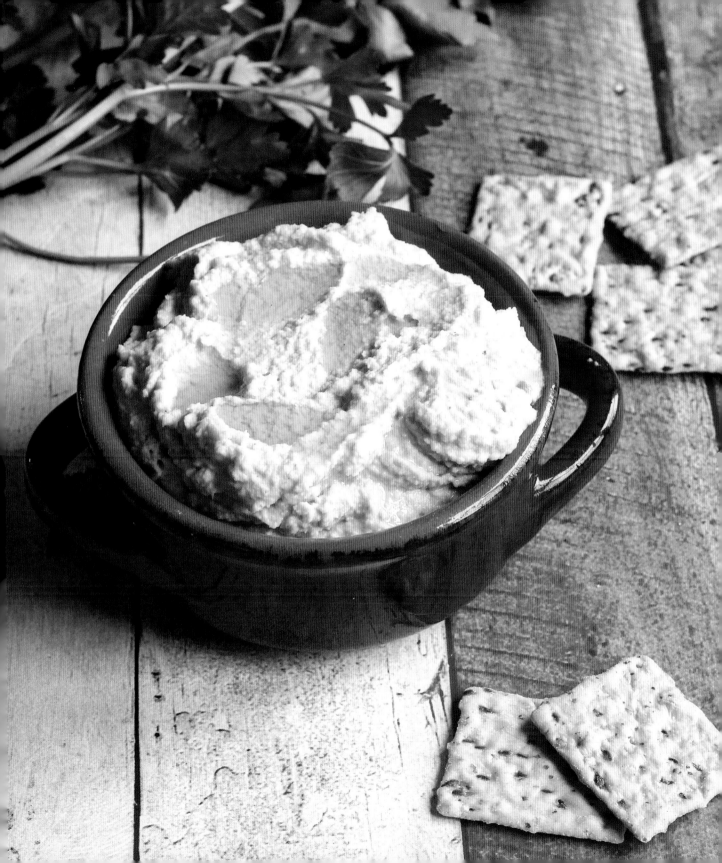

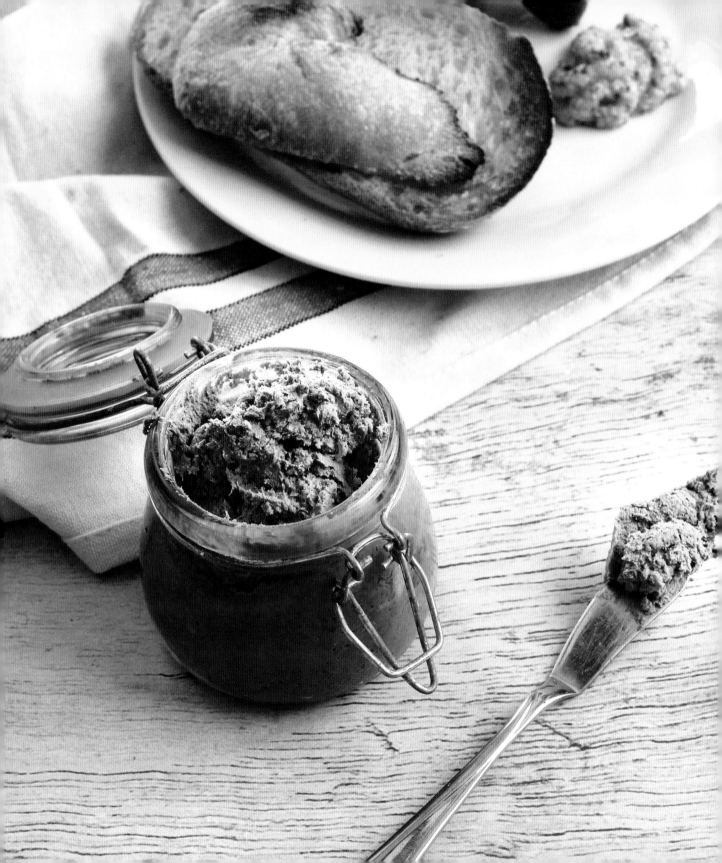

Organ meats in daily eating have nearly gone the way of the dinosaur. Modern palates and prudish attitudes about food have rendered organ meats, such as the heart, liver and kidneys, practically extinct from the average family's weekly menu. And we are seeing an unprecedented decline in hormonal health and fertility. Do you see the correlation? Because I do. Organ meats are the most nutrient-dense foods on the planet—with certain vitamins, such as vitamin B12, being present naturally in these meats.

Liver, in particular, is a valuable source of vitamins A, D and B12, as well as iron and selenium. These play an extremely important role in the production of reproductive and pituitary hormones. As such, eating liver is a major step in the direction of good hormonal health.

Grass-fed butter, apples, shallots and a bit of thyme transform duck or chicken liver into something remarkably delicious. Smeared on a crusty baguette and served with cornichons or capers, this pâté is a perfectly nutritious and indulgent meal.

BALANCING DUCK LIVER PÂTÉ

Flavor Profile: *Salty*

Serves: *4*

8 tbsp (112 g) butter, divided (4 tbsp [56 g] chilled)

1 large shallot, finely minced

1 small apple, peeled, cored and diced, such as a Golden Delicious

8 oz (226 g) duck or chicken livers, rinsed and drained

1 tsp fresh thyme leaves

1 tbsp (15 ml) Cognac (optional)

Salt & freshly ground pepper, to taste

In a skillet, melt 4 tablespoons (56 g) of butter over medium heat. Add the shallot and apple, and cook until they're translucent and softened, about 5 to 7 minutes. Add the livers and cook through, about 5 minutes. Remove it from the heat and allow it to cool for about 10 minutes.

Transfer the mixture to a food processor. Add the 4 tablespoons (56 g) of chilled butter, the thyme and Cognac, if using. Puree it until perfectly smooth. Season with salt and pepper to taste.

Place the pâté in a bowl or jar to serve, and chill it for at least 30 minutes or up to 3 to 4 days.

Herbalist Tip

Duck livers may be a little harder to find than chicken livers. If they are not available at your local grocer, most butchers will happily order them for you if you ask.

It is important to source pasture-raised, antibiotic-free, preferably organic livers whenever possible, as the liver can accumulate toxins.

Pumpkin seeds are not just for snacking after carving your Halloween pumpkin. As an herbalist, pumpkin seed infusions are one of my go-to remedies for prostate complaints.

Numerous studies show that pumpkin seeds and virgin pumpkin seed oil promote prostate health and help mitigate the symptoms of prostate enlargement, such as frequent urination, weak stream and difficulty starting and stopping urination. It is estimated that as many as 50 percent of men ages 51 to 60 suffer from this frustrating and embarrassing condition. Lime and cayenne pepper are inflammation fighters that promote good circulation, greatly benefiting prostate health. Who knew that relieving this condition could be as simple as eating a couple palmfuls of these delicious, spicy little seeds every day!

Pumpkin seeds are extremely high in zinc which helps in matters of immunity, stress tolerance, anxiety and concentration. Other studies indicate that pumpkin seeds may help to correct male pattern baldness that occurs in both men AND women due to high androgenic hormones associated with aging.

LIME & CHILE PUMPKIN SEEDS

Flavor Profile: *Sweet, Salty, Sour*
Makes: *2 cups (280 g)*

2 cups (280 g) raw pumpkin seeds (whole or shelled)

1 tbsp (15 ml) virgin pumpkin seed oil

1 tbsp (15 ml) fresh lime juice

1 tsp freshly grated lime zest

Pinch to ¼ tsp cayenne pepper, or more to taste

½ tsp fine sea salt

Preheat your oven to 325°F (170°C, or gas mark 3). Line a rimmed baking sheet with parchment paper.

In a small bowl, toss the raw pumpkin seeds and pumpkin seed oil until the seeds are evenly coated. Place the coated seeds on the lined baking sheet. Roast for 40 to 50 minutes, tossing or stirring occasionally or until the seeds produce a nutty aroma and are very lightly toasted.

Remove the baking sheet from the oven and place the seeds in a small bowl. Immediately toss the warm seeds with the lime juice, lime zest, cayenne pepper and sea salt. Place the seeds back on the lined baking sheet. Return it to the oven for 5 to 10 minutes, or until the seeds are dry.

Remove the baking sheet from the oven and cool the seeds completely on the tray. Transfer to a container with an airtight lid and store in a cool, dry place.

Herbalist Tip
This recipe can be made with either whole or shelled seeds. Eating whole seeds increases the fiber content, but may cause digestive discomforts for certain sensitive individuals.

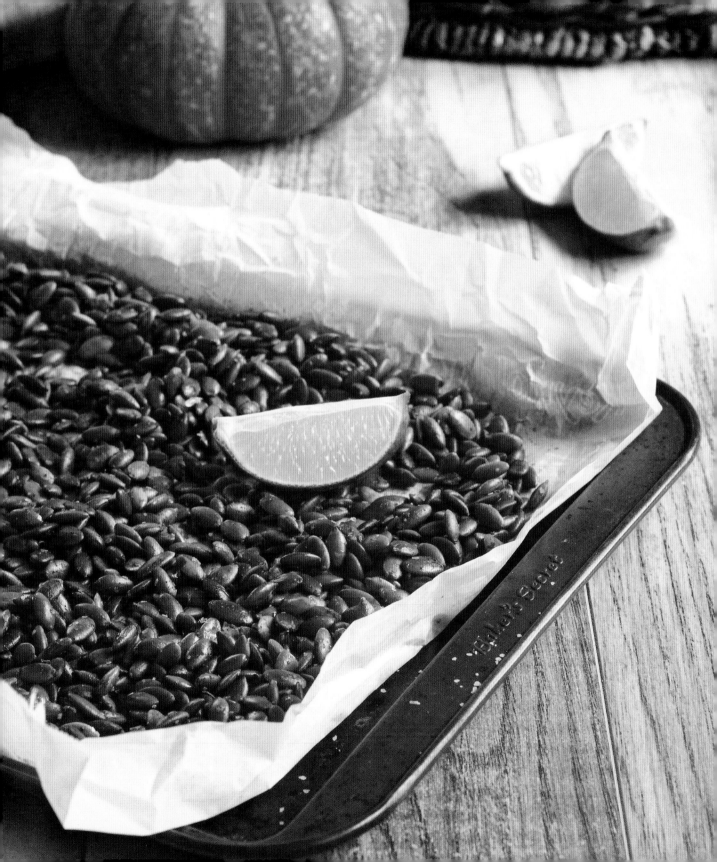

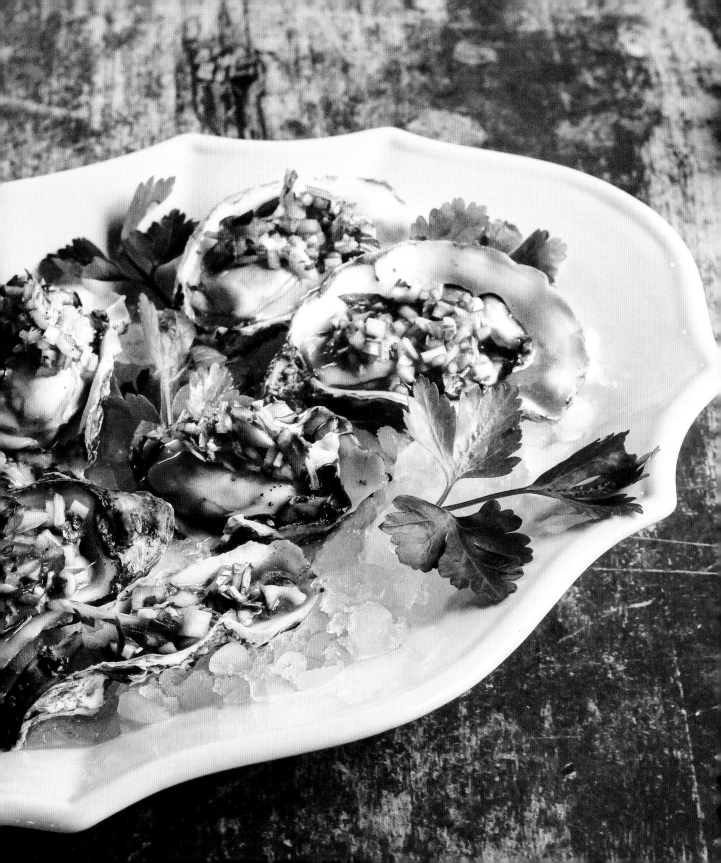

As a seafood lover and with seafaring in my blood, eating raw oysters on the half shell is a much-anticipated event. Oysters are a special treat that I greatly enjoy, but raw oysters give some folks the heebie-jeebies. They are cold and slippery. You don't really want to chew them a whole lot. I get it. But oysters are oh-so-very good for you.

Oysters have a reputation as an aphrodisiac. But did you know that they are loaded, I mean *loaded*, with minerals such as zinc, iron and selenium that support reproductive and adrenal health? They are an excellent source of vitamins A, C, E and the elusive B12. Oysters also encourage good cardiovascular health and blood flow—perhaps nodding to the ole libido-boosting benefits.

Serve this dish chilled with a generous spoonful of tangy sauce for garnish. My mignonette sauce contains detoxifying parsley and cycle-regulating tarragon for added herbal health benefits.

OYSTERS ON THE HALF SHELL WITH MIGNONETTE SAUCE

Flavor Profile: *Salty, Pungent*
Serves: *2*

12 petite whole oysters, scrubbed and shucked

Crushed, salted ice

⅓ cup (80 ml) red wine vinegar

2 large shallots, minced

1 tbsp (5 g) minced parsley

1 tbsp (4 g) tarragon

½ –1 tsp freshly ground pepper

Sea salt, to taste

Gently loosen the oysters from their shells, keeping as much oyster liquor in the shells with the oysters as possible. Place them on a rimmed tray lined with crushed, salted ice.

In a small bowl, whisk together the vinegar, shallots, parsley, tarragon, pepper and salt to taste. Spoon the sauce over the chilled oysters. Serve immediately.

Herbalist Tip
It is said that oysters should only be eaten in months containing the letter "R." I consider oysters a rare winter treat that should be sourced from cool and clean waters.

I promised that this book would contain everyday foods and herbs, but there are a few recipes that reach for the exotic and the wild. And I can think of no better place to use those sexy ingredients than in these sensuous, aphrodisiac hand-rolled truffles.

Rose has been associated with love and romance since time immemorial. The alluring aroma of the flower queen and her characteristic floral flavor offer these truffles a sexy veil of botanical goodness. *Maca*, also known as Peruvian ginseng, is a root that is traditionally used to support energy and fertility and to encourage a robust libido. Chocolate, here in the form of roasted cacao and dark chocolate, is also considered an aphrodisiac. These truffles are sure to ignite the passionate fires within, and they are the perfect end to a romantic meal.

ROSE & MACA HAND-ROLLED TRUFFLES

Flavor Profile: *Bitter, Sweet*
Makes: *40 to 60 truffles*

½ cup (120 ml) heavy cream

2 tbsp (28 g) butter

2 tsp (14 g) honey or maple syrup

2 tbsp (30 g) maca powder

8 oz (226 g) good-quality dark chocolate, finely chopped

For Rolling

⅓ cup (32 g) roasted cacao powder

1 cup (15 g) dried rose petals, powdered

2 tbsp (20 g) dried beet root powder

Set up a double boiler over gently simmering water; make sure that the top bowl is not in contact with the water. Add the heavy cream, butter, honey, maca powder and dark chocolate. Stir until they're melted and remove the bowl from the heat as soon as the mixture is smooth and shiny, about 4 to 5 minutes. DO NOT overheat as this will result in a grainy truffle. In fact, you can often pull your chocolate off the heat before everything is completely melted and stir until it's smooth.

Refrigerate for at least 30 to 40 minutes until the mixture is firm, but still scoop-able. While the chocolate is chilling, place the roasted cacao powder in a small bowl and combine the powdered rose petals and beet root powder in another. Line a baking sheet with parchment paper.

When the chocolate mixture is chilled, scoop it using a tablespoon and roll it into ½- to 1-inch (1.3- to 2.5-cm) balls, then roll each truffle in either the cacao or rose–beet root powder. Place the truffles on the lined baking tray and store them in a cool spot or refrigerate. Allow the truffles to come to room temperature for about 30 minutes before serving.

Herbalist Tips
Maca, rose petals and beet root powder may be difficult to find in a standard grocery store, but are available at well-stocked herb stores and from online retailers.

You can grind the rose petals to a fine powder by using a dedicated coffee grinder, food processor or mortar and pestle.

Roll half of these truffles in roasted cacao powder and the other half in rose and beet root powder for a visually stunning presentation.

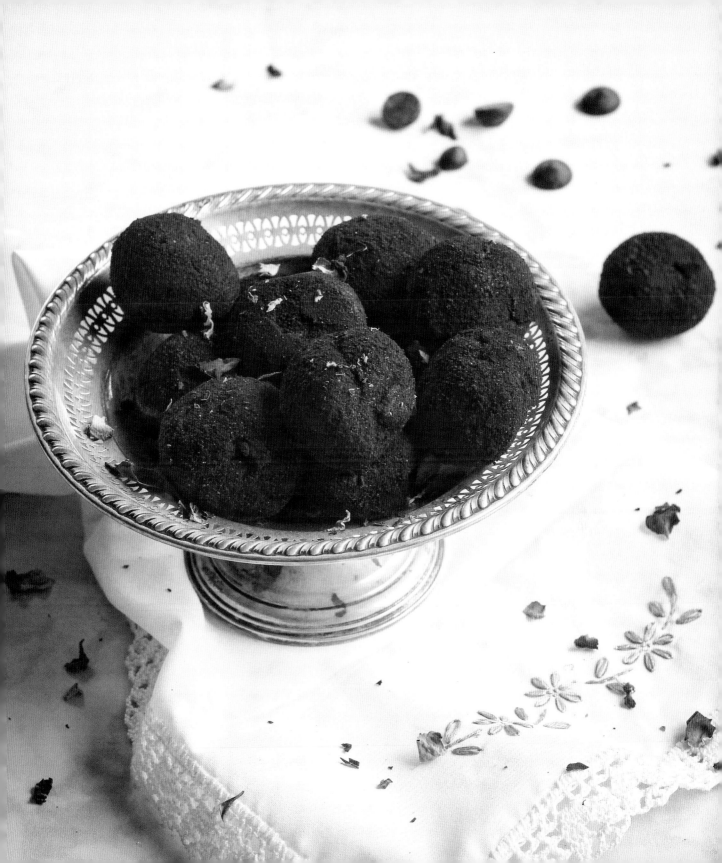

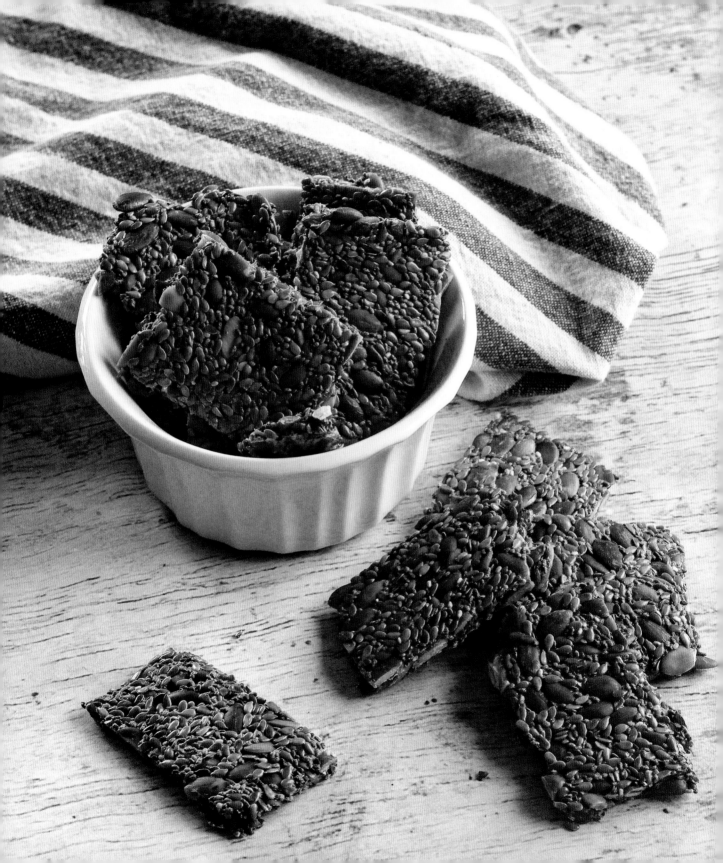

Women who suffer with hormonal imbalance and infertility might have heard about a process called seed cycling or seed rotation. The theory behind it holds that certain seeds contain the proteins, fibers and phytonutrients to encourage hormonal health. In seed cycling, flax and pumpkin seeds are encouraged during the follicular phase (days 1 to 14 of your cycle). Sesame and sunflower seeds are suggested during the luteal phase (days 14 to 28). The follicular-phase seeds promote estrogen production, followed by progesterone encouraged by the luteal-phase seeds.

Ladies experiencing irregular cycles, cramping, cysts and infertility may find a return to a more normal cycle and increased fertility by practicing consistent seed cycling. These crackers were made to maximize the amount of seeds consumed daily; it is suggested that one consume 2 tablespoons (15 g) each day. I add red raspberry leaf and a pinch of ginger to this tasty, protein-rich snack to create even more reproductive-system love!

SEED CYCLING CRACKERS

Flavor Profile: *Sweet*

Makes: *2 sheet trays of crackers*

1½ cups (252 g) flaxseeds (follicular) or sunflower seeds (luteal)

1½ cups (210 g) pumpkin seeds (follicular) or sesame seeds (luteal)

½ cup (88 g) chia seeds

1 tsp salt

2 tbsp (18 g) dried red raspberry leaf

1 tsp ground ginger

1½ cups (355 ml) water

Preheat your oven to 350°F (175°C, or gas mark 4).

Mix the follicular- or luteal-phase seeds with the chia, salt, raspberry leaf and ginger. Add the water and soak them for 10 to 15 minutes, until the mixture is thick and pasty.

Line two rimmed baking sheets with parchment paper or silicone mats. Spread the mixture evenly to about ⅛ inch (3 mm) in each.

Bake for 1 hour, rotating the trays after 30 minutes, or until golden and crisp.

Remove the trays from the oven. If you desire a uniform cracker, score them while still warm to the desired shape and size. Cool them completely on the baking sheets and break them when they've cooled. Store them in an airtight container for up to 2 weeks.

I have had a lifelong love affair with citrus. Send me all the citrus. Send me all the sour. And I find this zingy citrus curd an especially pleasing treat.

Though lemon curd is more common, this grapefruit curd is delicious. Grapefruit is known for its wonderful benefits for immunity. High-lycopene foods, such as red and pink grapefruit, peaches, tomatoes and red peppers, are also associated with a decreased risk of prostate cancer! An addition of rose hips adds another layer of antioxidant action to this recipe.

Try this grapefruit curd on toasted English muffins or spooned atop a light angel food cake.

ZINGY GRAPEFRUIT & ROSE HIP CURD

Flavor Profile: *Sour*

Makes: *About 2 cups (450 g)*

6 egg yolks

¾ cup (175 ml) fresh grapefruit juice

2 tbsp (12 g) grapefruit zest

¾ cup (150 g) sugar

½ cup (112 g) butter

1 tbsp (8 g) dried rose hips

Place the egg yolks, grapefruit juice, zest, sugar, butter and rose hips in a small saucepan. Over medium-low heat, stirring constantly, cook until the mixture thickens, about 30 minutes. A whisk moving through the mixture should leave a noticeable trace. The curd will continue to thicken upon cooling

When the grapefruit mixture is thickened, remove it from the heat and pass it through a fine-mesh sieve into a bowl to remove the zest and any cooked egg. Place a layer of parchment or plastic film directly on the warm curd to prevent a crust from forming. Refrigerate until the curd is cold, about 4 to 6 hours.

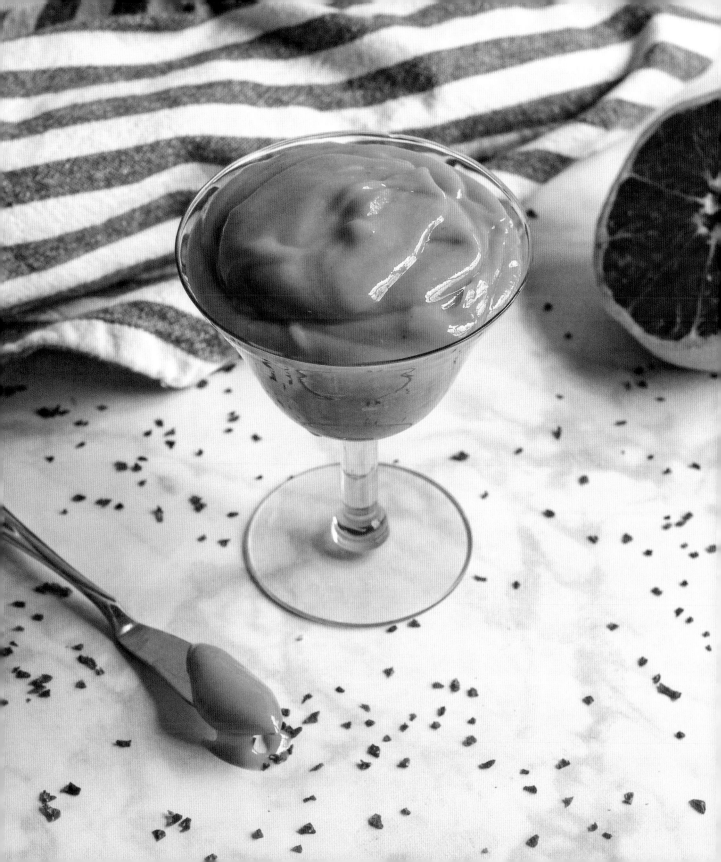

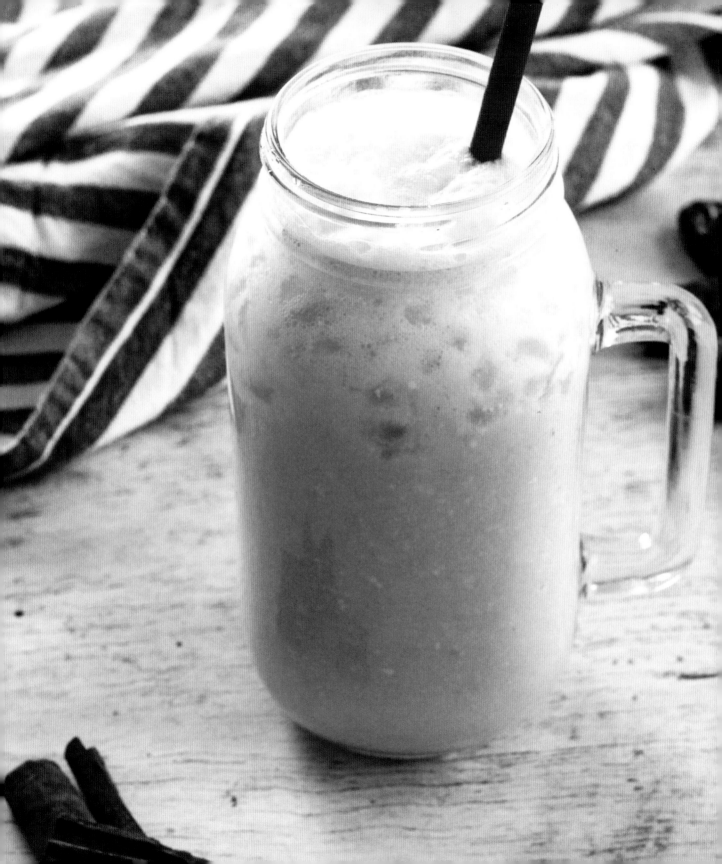

My first experience with *horchata* was a rush of intoxicating sweetness that nearly knocked me off my feet. . . . I wanted to love it, but it was so cloyingly sweet that my taste buds and my brain could not handle the sugar overload. With reports of obesity, infertility and hormonal imbalance on the rise, there is no question that we should curb our consumption of processed and added sugars. Insulin resistance is one of the chief causes of hormonal imbalance and infertility, so our food choices have a direct and immediate effect on reproductive health.

This recipe is sweetened with fiber- and potassium-rich dates and flavored with true cinnamon (*Cinnamomum zeylanicum*). True cinnamon, also called Ceylon cinnamon, is a potent hypoglycemic agent helping to decrease insulin resistance and prevent spikes in blood glucose. This dairy-free and hormone-healthy version of horchata is sure to delight.

DATE-SWEETENED CINNAMON HORCHATA

Flavor Profile: *Sweet, Pungent*
Makes: *About ½ gallon (1.9 L)*

6 cups (1.4 L) water, divided

¾ cup (140 g) long-grain white rice

2 whole Ceylon cinnamon sticks

½–¾ cup (89–134 g) pitted dates

1½ tsp (8 ml) pure vanilla extract

1 cup (235 ml) full-fat unsweetened coconut milk

Ice, for serving

Boil 2 cups (475 ml) of water, then pour it over the rice. Soak the rice for about 2 hours.

Crush the cinnamon sticks by placing them in a plastic bag or in a soft lint-free cloth. Then pound them with a mallet until they are broken into small pieces, about ¼ inch (6 mm) or smaller.

Drain the rice. Add it to a blender with the remaining 4 cups (940 ml) of water, the dates and vanilla. Blend them on high for 1 to 2 minutes. Transfer it to a jar and add the crushed cinnamon sticks. Place a lid on the jar and allow the mixture to stand in the refrigerator for at least 12 hours.

After 12 hours, strain the mixture through several layers of cheesecloth. Bundle the cloths and squeeze it to extract all the liquid. Whisk the coconut milk into the rice "milk" until well homogenized.

Pour the mixutre over ice and enjoy. Extra horchata can be stored in the refrigerator for up to 1 week.

Herbalist Tips
You can adjust the sweetness of the horchata by increasing the dates.

Make sure to use full-fat coconut milk, as it adds a lovely richness to this horchata.

True cinnamon, *Cinnamomum zeylanicum*, can be found in well-stocked herb stores or from online retailers.

It might come as a complete surprise to some, but goji berries are strongly linked to male reproductive health. Studies have linked higher testosterone production and increased fertility in both diabetic rats and those with late-onset hypogonadism. Both studies offer great insight into naturally treating male sexual dysfunction.

Smoothies are a simple and effective way to deliver nutrient-dense calories. This smoothie isn't just for men; it offers cardiovascular benefits and an excellent vitamin profile. It's made with milk kefir for its complex probiotic content, but you could substitute yogurt or nut milks.

GOJI BERRY & STRAWBERRY SMOOTHIE

Flavor Profile: *Sour, Sweet*
Serves: *2*

2 tbsp (20 g) dried goji berries

1 cup (145 g) fresh strawberries, hulled

2 cups (475 ml) milk kefir, yogurt or nut milk

1 cup (240 g) crushed ice

Honey, to taste

Add the goji berries to a small bowl and cover them with water. Soak the berries for at least 20 minutes to soften them.

Drain the goji berries. Add them to a blender with the strawberries, kefir and ice. Blend on high until it's perfectly smooth, about 30 seconds. Taste for sweetness and add a small amount of honey to taste, then blend until it's incorporated.

Pour the smoothie into chilled glasses and serve immediately.

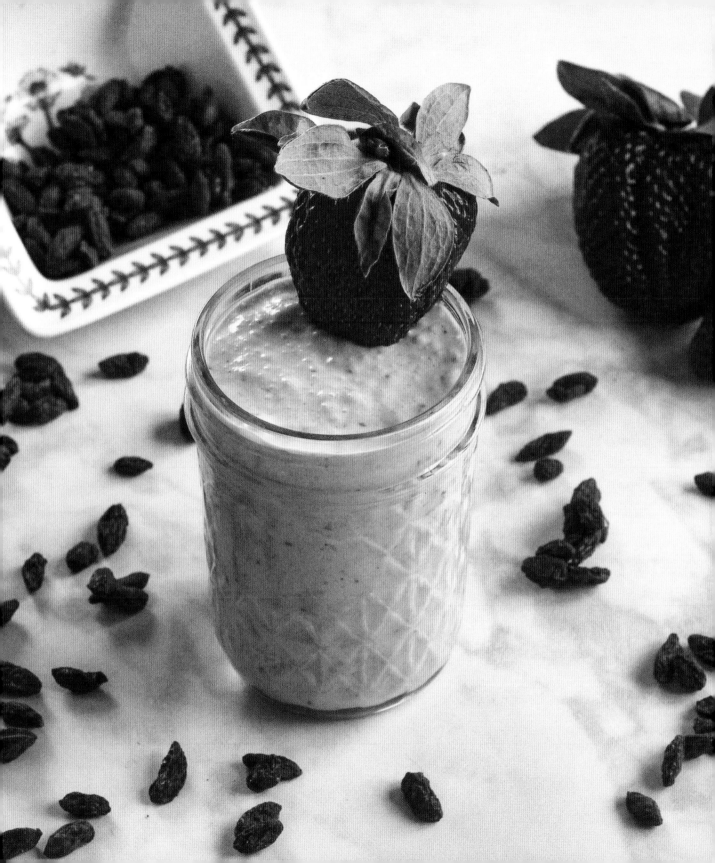

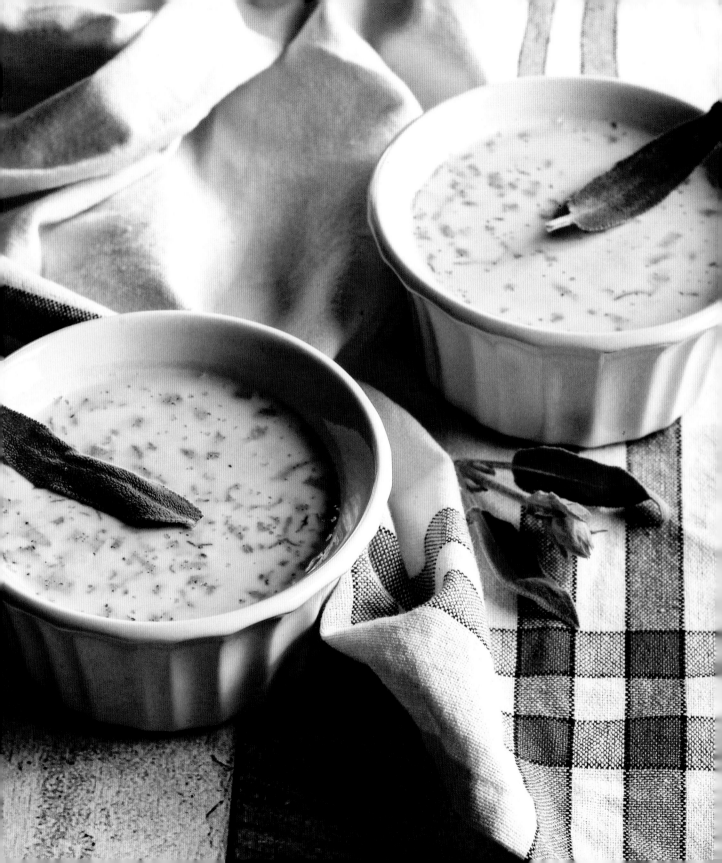

Puddings don't have to be for dessert. They can be savory. And, they can be medicinal. This panna cotta is just that: savory and medicinal.

Pumpkin serves as a fantastic base; it is easy to digest and moist with cooling properties. Sage is a profoundly cooling herb. And panna cotta is served chilled. All totaled, this is the perfect dish to fight some of the more irritating aspects of menopause such as hot flashes and dryness.

Serve as an appetizer for a fall dinner party or as a side dish anytime.

SAVORY PUMPKIN-SAGE PANNA COTTA

Flavor Profile: *Bitter, Sweet*

Serves: *4 to 6*

1 (0.25-oz [7-g]) envelope unflavored gelatin

1½ cups (355 ml) milk, divided

1 cup (235 ml) heavy cream

1 cup (245 g) pureed pumpkin or squash

1 tbsp (3 g) minced fresh sage leaves

Salt & freshly ground pepper, to taste

In a medium-sized bowl, sprinkle the packet of gelatin over ½ cup (120 ml) of milk and allow it to bloom for about 10 minutes.

Add the heavy cream and pumpkin. Whisk until it's completely smooth, about 30 to 60 seconds; you may need to blend the mixture in a blender to get it perfectly smooth.

In a small saucepan, add the remaining milk and sage. Bring it to a simmer over medium heat just until steam starts to rise, about 3 to 5 minutes. Remove the pan from the heat. Whisk the milk mixture into the pumpkin mixture. Taste for seasoning and add salt and pepper to taste.

Pour it into four to six individual serving bowls or ramekins. Chill the panna cotta in the refrigerator for 4 to 6 hours until it's set. Serve chilled.

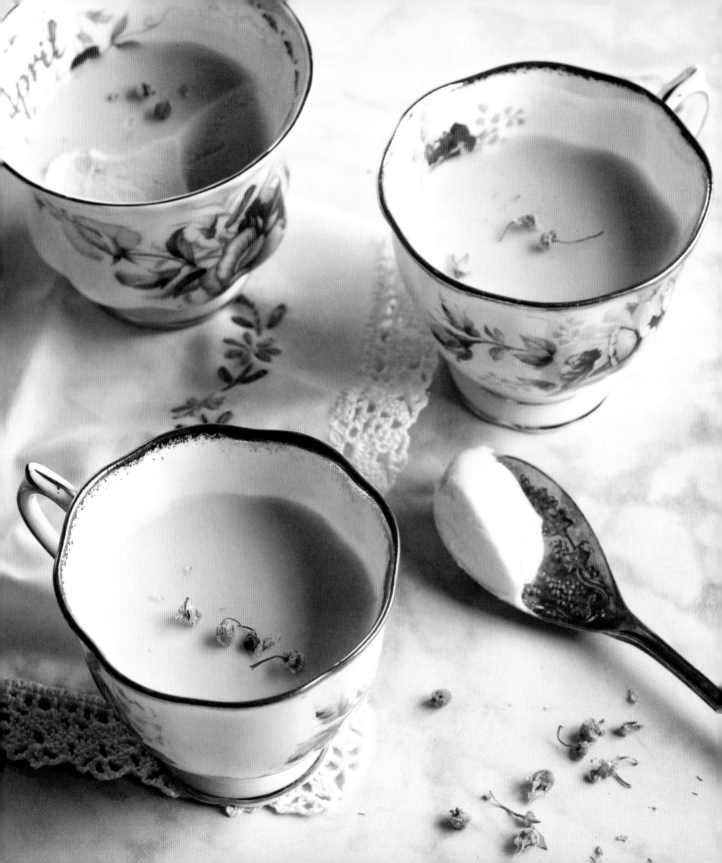

SEVEN

RECIPES TO

KEEP YOUR SKIN, BONES & MUSCLES IN TIP-TOP SHAPE

Health class taught us that a varied and nutrient-rich diet will help us to grow strong and tall. But did anybody tell us how to make this a reality? Not so much!

Fortification sounds profoundly militaristic, but when we are building the complex cellular matrix that is our skin, bones and muscles, fortifying foods are exactly what we need. We need to look to nutrient-dense foods with a diverse array of vitamins, minerals and phytonutrients that will offer the building blocks both for growth and for cellular repair.

The flavor profiles that often contain these vital materials are the much misunderstood sweet and salty. Body-building herbs—such as alfalfa, nettle and even chamomile— offer minerals essential to building and maintaining a healthy body. Pungent herbs such as cumin and cayenne maximize the absorption of various nutrients.

Ladle up a bowl of Bone Broth with Bone-Building Herbs (page 148) to replenish spent mineral stores. Bite into a flaky, stinging nettle–filled Spanakopita Triangle (page 156) for a foraging spin on a Greek classic. Or try a delicate, smooth Chamomile Posset (page 151) so full of calcium that your bones will thank you for days.

Do your body a solid and start cooking with intention. Your food choices will keep you strong.

Farm wives have been making bone broth for years in the "waste not, want not" way of life. Using every part of a harvested animal keeps your family fed and is respectful of the life that was sacrificed for nourishment. This recipe uses peeled chicken feet for a thick, silky broth; they can be ordered from your grocery store butcher. If you are uncomfortable with chicken feet, wing tips can also be ordered from the butcher.

Bone broth is a nutritious food that offers tremendous benefits. The minerals and collagen that are extracted over the course of hours or days make for a nutrient-dense broth. The broth is full of vital amino acids that support bone and connective tissue health as well as skin firmness and elasticity. Bone broths are ideal for those with a delicate digestive system as the gelatin present in the broth helps to repair the mucosal lining of the GI tract. Robust herbs such as stinging nettle and clover contribute vitamins and minerals vital to cellular growth and repair.

Bone broth will be quite gelatinous when cool. This contributes a silky texture when used in soups and stews.

BONE BROTH WITH BONE-BUILDING HERBS

Flavor Profile: *Salty*

Makes: *A generous gallon (3.8 L)*

1–1½ lb (450–680 g) bones from a whole chicken

½ lb (226 g) peeled and washed chicken feet or wing tips

2 ribs celery, roughly chopped

2 large carrots, roughly chopped

1 large onion, roughly chopped

2–3 cloves garlic, smashed

2 tbsp (30 ml) apple cider vinegar

¼ cup (7 g) dried nettle leaves

¼ cup (7 g) dried red clover blossoms

Salt & freshly ground pepper, to taste

Add the bones, feet, celery, carrots, onion, garlic, vinegar, nettle, clover blossoms and salt and pepper, to taste, to a large stockpot or slow cooker. Add enough cold water to cover the chicken carcass by about 3 to 4 inches (7.5 to 10 cm). Bring it to a gentle simmer and cook, covered, for a minimum of 12 hours, up to 36 hours.

After simmering the stock, strain it through several layers of cheesecloth or flour sack cloth. Pour the stock into quart- or pint-sized (940- or 475-ml) containers, leaving room for expansion, and freeze them. Alternatively, this bone broth can be pressure-canned; do not water-bath can this broth. Note: The high temperatures will affect its ability to properly gel when cooled.

Herbalist Tip
Bone broth should never be aggressively boiled. Maintain a gentle simmer for long periods of time to ensure a clear, rich broth.

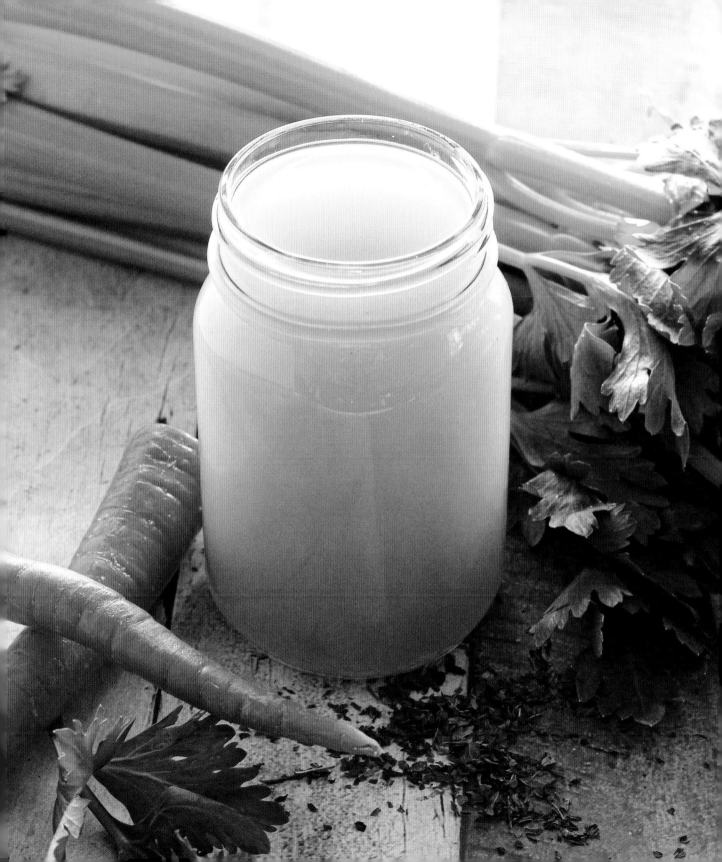

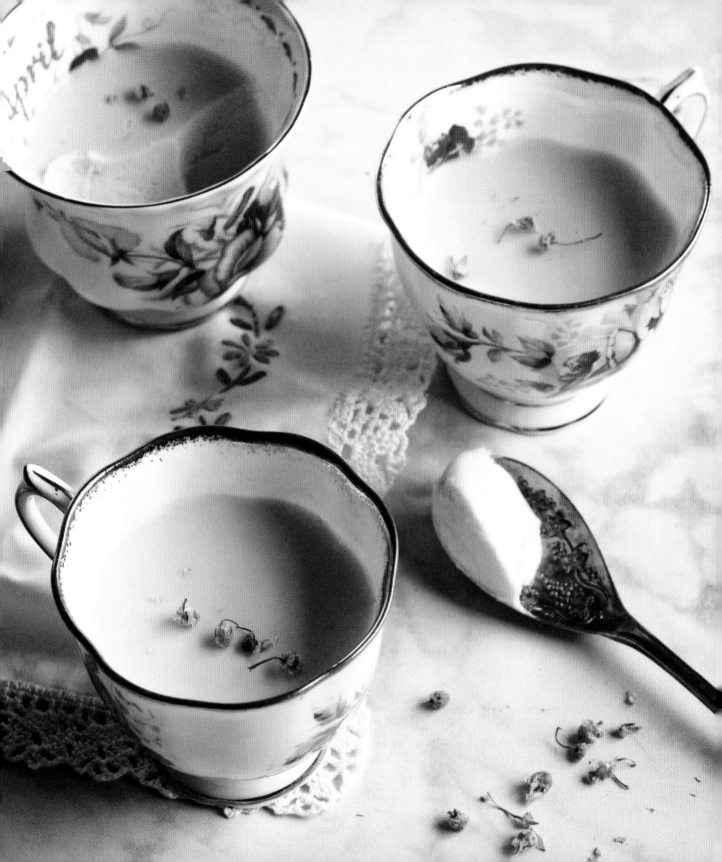

What is a posset? It is a pudding-like concoction of heavy cream, honey and lemon juice that is simmered and then chilled until set. I was first introduced to possets when my friend Danielle from Gather.com presented an oh-so-lovely version of the classic posset infused with delicate and ephemeral lilac flowers. As a sucker for all things floral and all things custard, I was transfixed.

This posset is infused with a favorite medicinal herb: chamomile. The soft floral and apple-like aroma of dried chamomile flowers perfumes and flavors this posset in the most magical way. While the posset is rich and creamy, the aromatics of the chamomile offer levity and brightness.

You might be surprised to find out chamomile is full of calcium and magnesium, making this dessert excellent for fortifying bones and relieving musculoskeletal pain. I make this posset now for my youngest daughter who is plagued with growing pains that trouble her muscles and bones.

CHAMOMILE POSSET

Flavor Profile: *Sweet*

Serves: *4 to 6*

4 cups (940 ml) heavy or whipping cream

¼ cup (8 g) dried chamomile flowers, or 8–10 chamomile tea bags

½ cup (170 g) raw honey

½ cup (120 ml) fresh lemon juice

Fresh or dried chamomile flowers, for garnish

In a small saucepan, add the heavy cream and chamomile. Bring it to a simmer over medium-low heat. When the cream has been brought to a simmer, reduce the heat to low and simmer for 5 minutes. Remove the pan from the heat. Cool the cream for at least 20 minutes or refrigerate for up to 24 hours.

Strain away the chamomile flowers. Add the infused cream along with the honey to a small saucepan. Over medium heat, stirring constantly, bring the mixture to a gentle simmer. Reduce the heat to maintain a very gentle simmer—do not boil. Cook and stir for 3 minutes.

Remove it from the heat and stir in the lemon juice. Pour the hot mixture into individual serving dishes. Chill for at least 24 hours until the posset is set. Garnish with one or two chamomile flowers and serve chilled.

With this Green Bean Confit, a simple vegetable gets a gorgeous transformation and a spotlight shining on its amazing health benefits. Caramelized onions and green beans simmer in a bath of peppery olive oil until they are buttery and tender. Then they're served with a splash of balsamic vinegar and a pinch of red pepper flakes.

Lest you think that this is just a Cinderella makeover on an unsuspecting vegetable, I will fill you in on the best part. Green beans are full of minerals that promote strong bones, healthy muscles, great hair and youthful skin. They offer ample amounts of calcium, iron, magnesium and riboflavin, as well as vitamin K.

A tiny pinch of red pepper flakes in this recipe promotes digestion. A more generous amount will impart the anti-inflammatory properties of capsaicin to the dish, which may help to relieve inflammation due to injury or stress.

GREEN BEAN CONFIT

Flavor Profile: *Salty, Pungent*

Serves: *4 to 6*

1 medium onion, sliced pole to pole

½ cup (120 ml) extra-virgin olive oil, divided

4 cups (440 g) fresh or frozen and thawed green beans, cut to 1-inch (2.5-cm) length

2 tbsp (30 ml) balsamic vinegar

Salt & freshly ground pepper, to taste

Red pepper flakes, to taste

In a heavy-bottomed or cast-iron pan over medium-high heat, sauté the onion in 2 tablespoons (30 ml) of olive oil until it turns a deep golden color, about 20 minutes. Stir and adjust the temperature as needed so that the onion doesn't burn.

Add the remaining olive oil and the green beans, stirring them into the onions. Spread them evenly and place a second heavy pan on top of the mixture to weigh it down and create more contact with the bottom of the pan. Reduce the heat to medium. Cook for about 20 minutes, or until the bottom beans have browned and all the beans are tender.

Remove the pans from the heat and remove the pan used for weight. Toss the beans and onion with balsamic vinegar and season with salt, pepper and red pepper flakes to taste.

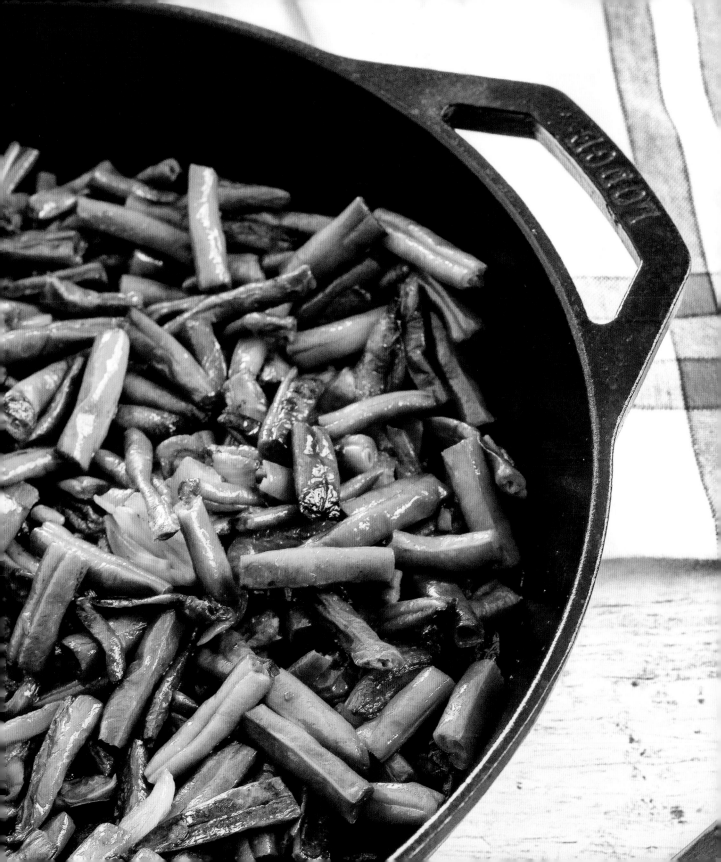

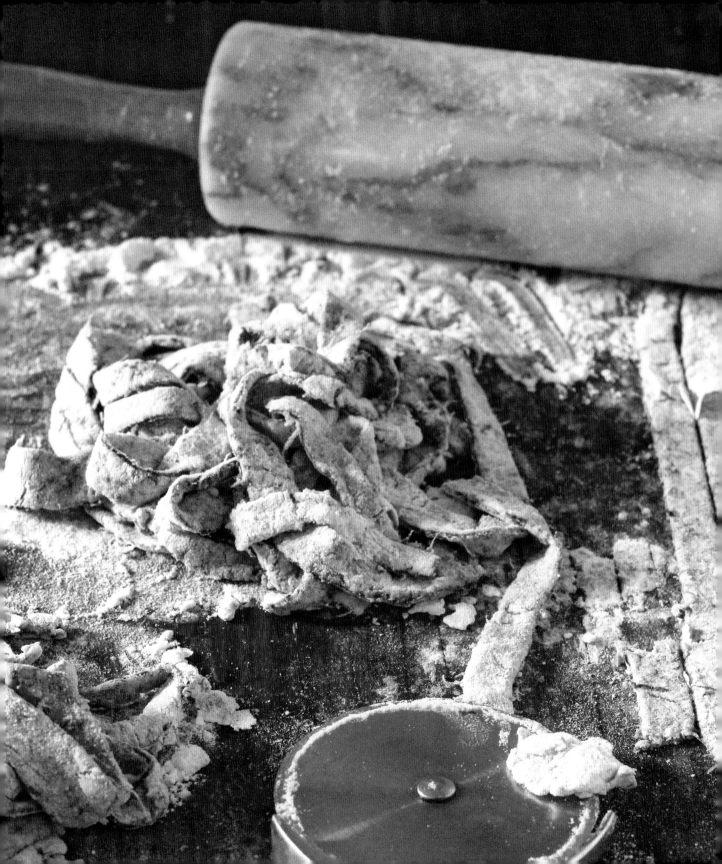

A fellow blogger, Kathie Lapcevic of Homespun Seasonal Living, created a batch of homemade egg noodles using dandelion—and I just knew that I had to do something similar with stinging nettle. If you have never had homemade egg noodles, you're in for a real treat. And freshly foraged stinging nettle delivers a punch of nutrition and earthy green flavor that is welcome on a late-winter day.

Nettle is a truly fortifying food, as well as one of my favorite medicinal herbs. It is high in vitamins A and K, loaded with calcium and manganese and full of quercetin, making it a highly restorative wild herb worth foraging for. In absence of fresh nettle, spinach may be substituted for a similar flavor and nutritional profile.

These noodles are best dressed simply with brown butter, toasted pine nuts and an aged hard cheese. Serve the noodles alone for a celebration of pasta, or alongside grilled chicken for a more substantial meal.

NETTLE EGG NOODLES

Flavor Profile: *Salty, Sweet*

Serves: *4 to 6*

4 cups (5 oz [142 g]) fresh stinging nettle leaves, packed

2 whole large eggs

2 cups (250 g) all-purpose flour, plus more if needed

½ tsp sea salt, plus more for pasta water

Your favorite sauce or brown butter and aged cheese, for serving

In a medium-sized saucepan, bring 6 cups (1.4 L) of water to a boil. Add the nettle and blanch them for 30 seconds. Strain the leaves and transfer them to an ice-water bath to shock. This process eliminates the sting of the nettle and preserves its bright green color.

Drain the nettle in a colander lined with cheesecloth and squeeze out any excess moisture. In a blender or a food processor, add the nettle and the eggs. Blend until it's smooth, about 20 to 30 seconds. Set it aside.

Sift together the flour and salt onto a clean work surface. Mound the flour mixture and make a well in the center. Pour the egg mixture into the well. Using a fork, work the flour into the liquid, about 5 minutes. You may need to add or subtract flour to achieve a slightly stiff dough.

When the dough is stiff, knead it on a floured work surface until it's smooth and elastic, about 3 to 5 minutes. Using a rolling pin or a pasta roller, roll the dough until it is about ⅛ inch (3 mm) thick. Using a pizza wheel or the cutting attachment on the pasta roller, cut to the desired length and width. Leave the pasta on the floured surface to rest.

Fill a large stockpot with water and a generous amount of salt. Place it over high heat and bring the water to a boil. When the water comes to a full boil, add the pasta. Cook for 5 to 7 minutes, until it's al dente, then strain. Do not rinse.

Dress the pasta with your favorite sauce, or with a little brown butter and aged cheese.

Spanakopita can be best described as a pie of greens with a little bit of cheese. I make mine with wilted greens, cheese and just a little lemon zest to bring some brightness to the filling that is sandwiched between buttery, flaky layers of fillo.

I love using spring stinging nettle, but spinach is an equally excellent source of vitamins, minerals and phytonutrients. Combined with feta and ricotta, this is a meal full of the calcium and magnesium that one needs to keep bones strong, healthy and pain-free!

SPANAKOPITA TRIANGLES

Flavor Profile: *Salty*

Makes: *12 parcels*

3 eggs, divided

2 cups (6 oz [170 g]) blanched or thawed stinging nettle or spinach, drained of excess liquid (see Herbalist Tip)

3 oz (85 g) ricotta cheese, drained of excess whey

8 oz (226 g) feta

Zest of 1 small lemon

Salt & freshly ground pepper

12 sheets of thawed fillo, wrapped in plastic or a slightly damp cloth to prevent drying out

½ cup (112 g) butter, melted

Preheat your oven to 350°F (175°C, or gas mark 4). Line a baking sheet with parchment paper.

In a small bowl, beat the eggs with a fork or a whisk for about 30 seconds. Remove a scant ¼ cup (60 ml) of the beaten eggs and set it aside. Combine the remaining eggs with the nettle, ricotta, feta and lemon zest, seasoning with salt and pepper to taste. Stir well and set it aside.

Brush 1 sheet of fillo pastry with butter, then add another layer of fillo. Repeat so that there are 3 layers of fillo and brush the top layer lightly with more butter. Cut the sheets into 3 long strips about 3 inches (7.5 cm) wide. Add 1 generous tablespoon (15 g) of filling at the end of each strip and fold it in "triangles" like a flag. Working quickly, repeat with the other sheets and filling until you have 12 filled fillo parcels.

Place the parcels on the lined baking sheet and brush them lightly with the reserved beaten egg. Bake until they're golden, about 20 to 22 minutes. Serve immediately.

Herbalist Tip

To blanch the stinging nettle, add the fresh leaves to a large pot of boiling water. Boil them for 20 to 30 seconds, then drain. After they have cooled for about 20 minutes, squeeze excess fluid from the leaves.

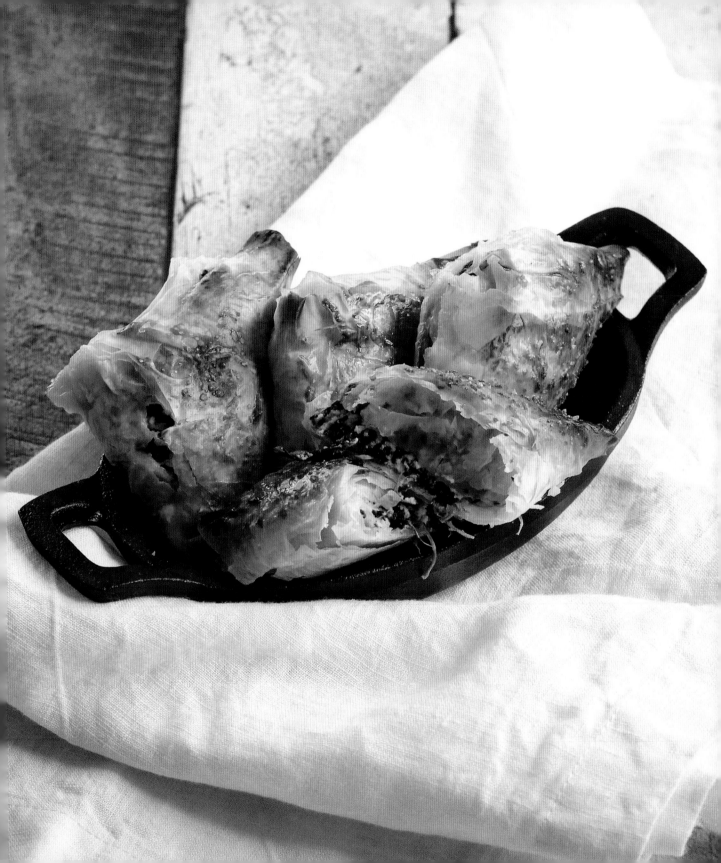

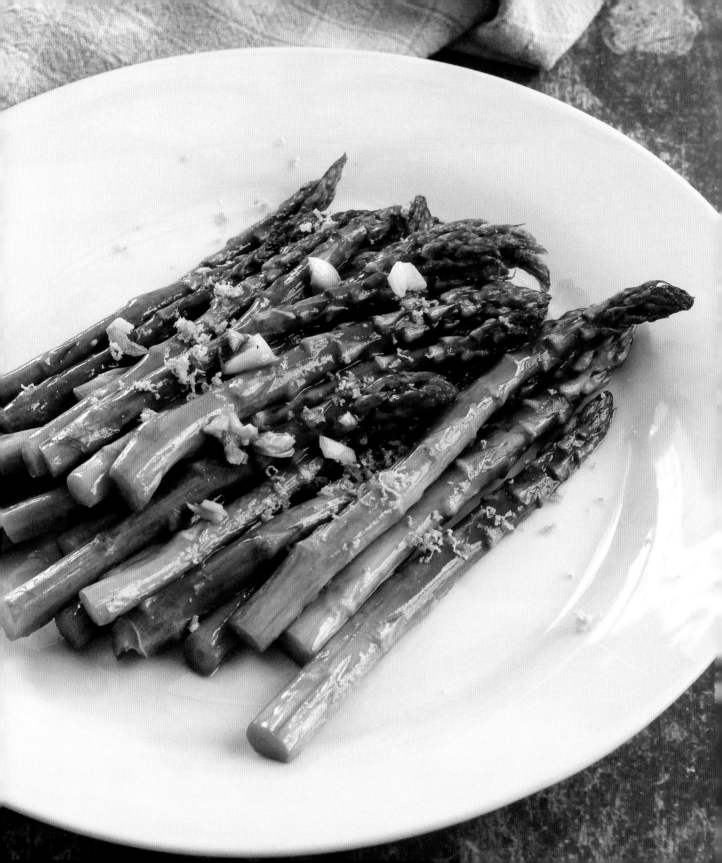

Asparagus is a wonderful example of food as medicine. These slender stalks are one of the most nutritionally balanced foods that one can consume. Asparagus stalks are especially high in glutathione which supports skin elasticity, prevents oxidative skin damage and visibly slows the signs of aging. And the benefits aren't just skin-deep; asparagus has folate—associated with reduced age-related cognitive decline. Additionally, the black pepper in the recipe adds profound anti-inflammatory benefits, which help us sidestep the damaging effects of inflammation in the skin tissues.

LEMONY PAN-ROASTED ASPARAGUS

Flavor Profile: *Salty, Bitter, Sour*

Serves: *4*

1 bunch asparagus spears, trimmed

2–3 cloves garlic, minced

3 tbsp (45 ml) extra-virgin olive oil

1 tsp sea salt

1 tsp ground black pepper

1 tbsp (15 ml) fresh lemon juice

Zest of 1 small lemon

Preheat your oven to 425°F (220°C, or gas mark 7).

Toss the asparagus and garlic with olive oil on a rimmed baking sheet. Roast for 10 to 15 minutes, until the spears start to brown very slightly around the edges.

Remove them from the oven. Add the salt, pepper, lemon juice and zest, and toss them well. Serve immediately.

Herbalist Tip

I love sturdy asparagus stalks for roasting. Avoid pencil-thin stalks and be sure to trim the stalks of woody ends.

Tikka masala is a warm, spicy and pungent Indian dish. The bold flavors and sweet spices are so satisfying. Traditionally it uses paneer, a fresh curd cheese, like ricotta, that is pressed, drained and cubed. However, I have found fresh mozzarella balls from my local cheese counter to be a clever and convenient substitute. The combination of mozzarella "paneer" and creamy Greek yogurt adds an indulgent texture and a mega-dose of calcium to this spicy dish! The spices of masala increase the digestive "fire," absorption and bioavailability of the phytonutrients, vitamins and minerals contained in the sauce. Paneer tikka masala is simply a dish that makes you feel stronger, replenished and fortified.

PRACTICAL "PANEER" TIKKA MASALA

Flavor Profile: *Sweet, Pungent, Sour*

Serves: *4 to 6*

Tikka Masala Spice Blend

2 tbsp (14 g) paprika

2 tbsp (12 g) ground coriander

2 tbsp (14 g) ground cumin

1 tsp ground pepper

1 tsp ground cardamom

1 tsp ground cinnamon

1 tsp ground turmeric

½–1½ tsp cayenne pepper, to taste

"Paneer" Tikka Masala

1 yellow onion, minced

2–3 cloves garlic, minced

1 tbsp (15 ml) extra-virgin olive oil

2–3 tbsp (20–30 g) tikka masala spice blend

1 (28-oz [794-g]) can fire roasted tomatoes

1 cup (200 g) plain Greek yogurt

8 oz (226 g) fresh mozzarella balls, halved or cubed to bite-size pieces

Sea salt, to taste

Cooked basmati rice, for serving

Cilantro, for garnish

To make the tikka masala spice blend, combine the paprika, coriander, cumin, pepper, cardamom, cinnamon, turmeric and cayenne pepper in a jar with a tight-fitting lid. Cover it with the lid and shake well to combine the spices.

To make the "paneer" tikka masala, in a large pan, sauté the onion and garlic in the olive oil over medium-high heat until they're translucent, about 5 to 7 minutes. Add the tikka masala blend to the cooked onion, and cook for about 1 to 2 minutes to "bloom" the spices. Add the tomatoes and stir well to combine them. Turn the heat to medium-low and simmer for 10 minutes.

After cooking, turn off the heat and add the Greek yogurt. Use an immersion blender to blend until it's smooth. Stir in the mozzarella and let it sit for 3 to 5 minutes to warm through. Season it with salt to taste. Serve over rice and garnish with cilantro.

Herbalist Tip

Store the unused portion of tikka masala blend in a lidded jar. Use it to flavor poultry, rice and grilled veggies!

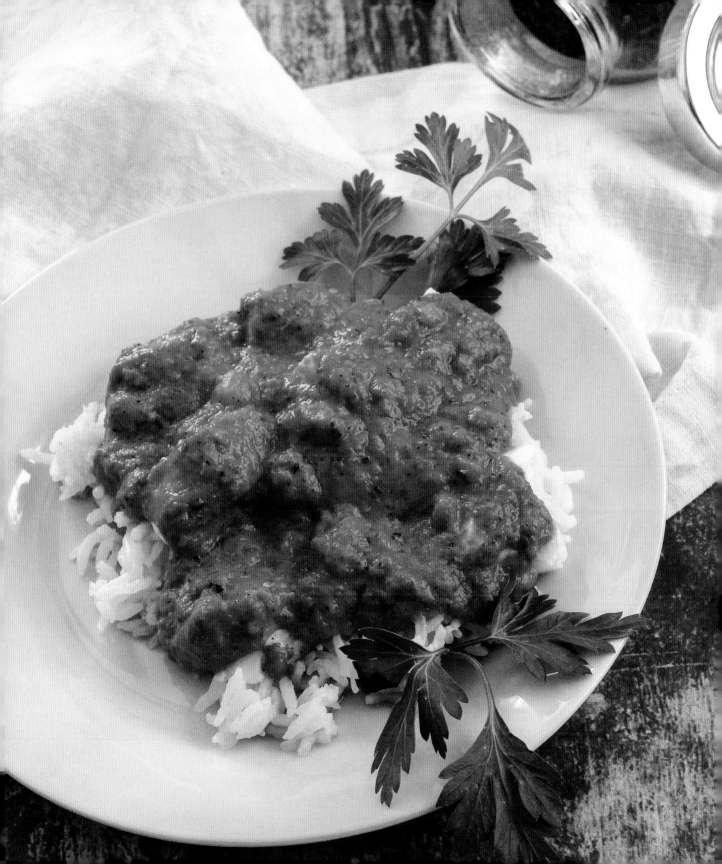

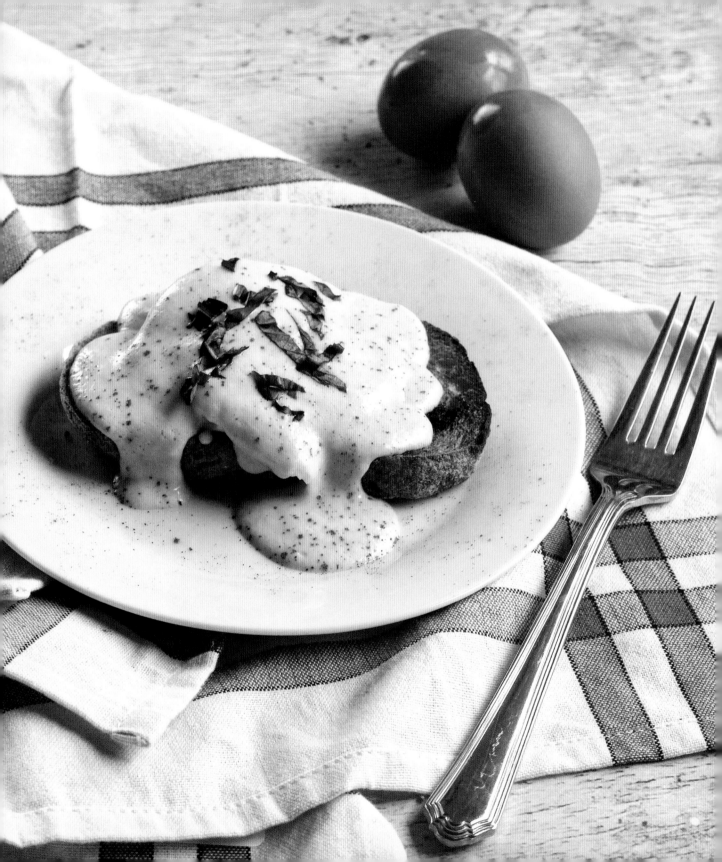

Eggs are fuel for the body and mind! In fact, they are one of the healthiest and most fortifying foods that we can consume. Research is finding that healthy fats, such as those found in eggs, offer many of the essential building blocks for cellular repair and for maintaining bones, muscles and skin—as well as nourishing the brain!

Hollandaise sauce is an emulsion-based sauce that requires a considerable skill to perfect. I recently learned a new technique involving room-temperature butter that makes this sauce positively foolproof!

Poached eggs with homemade hollandaise are typically served on a toasted English muffin with ham for eggs Benedict or cured salmon for eggs royale. I think it is delicious served over arugula and frisée. I added delicious fresh tarragon to the sauce; it lends a light licorice flavor, and it is associated with decreased pain from osteoarthritis. This dish offers so many of the vital nutrients to promote a healthy musculo-skeletal system and radiant skin!

POACHED EGGS WITH FOOLPROOF TARRAGON HOLLANDAISE

Flavor Profile: *Sweet, Salty*
Serves: *4 to 8*

Hollandaise Sauce
4 large egg yolks
8 tbsp (112 g) salted butter, softened
2 tsp (10 ml) fresh lemon juice
¼ tsp cayenne pepper or smoked paprika
1 tsp chopped tarragon

Poached Eggs
1 tbsp (15 ml) white vinegar
1 tsp sea salt
8 whole eggs

For Serving
English muffins, ham, salmon, arugula and frisée (optional)

For the hollandaise sauce, in a medium-sized heatproof bowl, add the egg yolks and butter. Place the bowl over a pan of barely simmering water, making sure that the bottom of the bowl is not touching the water. Gently whisk the eggs and softened butter while slowly pouring in ⅓ cup (80 ml) of hot water. Cook over the simmering water for about 7 to 10 minutes, or until the hollandaise sauce registers 160°F (71°C). Remove it from the heat and whisk in the lemon juice, cayenne and tarragon. Set aside.

To make the eggs, in a medium-sized pot with a lid, bring water to a boil. Add the vinegar and salt. Turn off the heat. Crack 4 eggs into a liquid measuring cup, and pour each egg out separately into the pot. Place a lid on the pot. Allow the eggs to cook in hot water for 3 minutes. Using a slotted spoon, remove the cooked eggs to a warm water bath. Return the pot to a boil; repeat the steps to cook the remaining 4 eggs.

To serve, remove the eggs and gently blot any excess water. Serve the eggs over your chosen medium and generously pour the hollandaise sauce over the eggs.

Herbalist Tip
Use the freshest eggs and butter from grass-fed cows for the most outstanding dish ever.

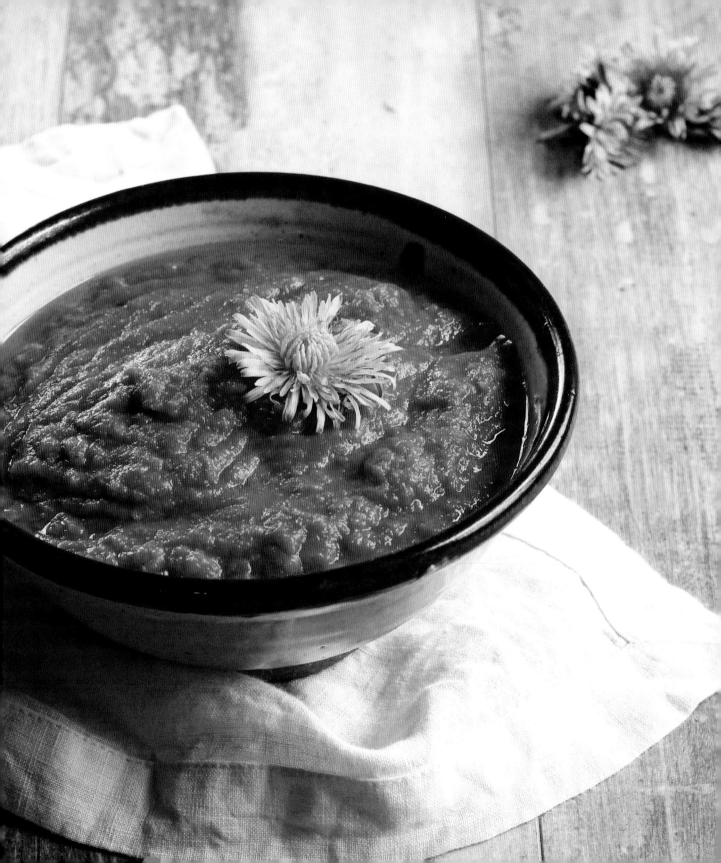

EIGHT

RECIPES TO

REJUVENATE YOUR MIND & SENSES

It's where the magic really, really happens: our central nervous system. But the part of our body that controls everything—the system that controls our thoughts and five senses—well, we don't think too much about nourishing that, now do we? When was the last time you thought about the foods that could support your eyesight, your memories and your every thought?

This final chapter of recipes to support the health of your mind and senses is perhaps the one that is dearest to me. If you've watched a loved one experience cognitive decline, experienced the loss or diminishment of one or more of your senses, or felt the inexplicable pain and disorientation of a misfiring nervous system, then you know just how frustrating these conditions are. Largely invisible to a bystander, matters of the mind and senses deserve to be treated with attention and care.

Let's talk brain food—or, more appropriately, central nervous system foods. The central nervous system craves soothing adaptogenic herbs such as basil, and it wants anti-inflammatory herbs such as turmeric to maintain focus and wellness. Let's use the twin powers of brainy Roasted Walnuts with Rosemary (page 173) for a snack you will surely remember. Maybe dip into the calming influences of basil with a Basil Cashew "Cheese" (page 166). And for a truly special treat, start your day with the ultimate indulgence—Mindful Hot Chocolate with Rhodiola (page 174).

Feed your senses. Invigorate your mind. Stimulate your soul.

Did you know that basil, the chief ingredient of pesto genovese and pizza alla margherita, is actually a profoundly brain-supportive herb? Culinary basil and its sister holy basil, also known as *tulsi*, are aromatic and adaptogenic herbs that favor good brain health. High in manganese, basil may increase neurotransmitter activity in the brain, improving cognition and stress response.

This recipe ups the healthy quotient with probiotics delivered by the whey or brine (see the Herbalist Tips), and it delivers cheesy flavor from the addition of nutritional yeast. My basil cashew "cheese" is a yummy treat spread on crackers or fresh vegetable slices.

The cashew cheese can also be loosened with pasta water and tossed with freshly cooked pasta for a light supper—or layer it into lasagna for an incredible, filling dinner.

BASIL CASHEW "CHEESE"

Flavor Profile: *Sweet, Salty*
Serves: *4 to 6*

2 cups (300 g) raw cashews, soaked in hot water for at least 20 minutes and drained

½ cup (120 ml) whey from drained yogurt, or brine from a vegetable ferment such as Daikon Radish Kimchi (page 61) or sauerkraut

2–3 cloves garlic, minced

¼ cup (20 g) nutritional yeast

1½ tbsp (25 ml) fresh lemon juice

1 cup (25 g) tightly packed fresh basil leaves (holy basil preferred)

Salt & freshly ground pepper, to taste

Place the drained cashews, whey, garlic, nutritional yeast, lemon juice and basil in the bowl of a food processor. Puree on high until it's perfectly smooth, about 2 to 3 minutes. Season with salt and pepper to taste.

At this point the "cheese" has a looser consistency. To achieve a texture more like that of fresh goat cheese, scoop the cashew cheese onto 2 to 3 layers of cheesecloth and tie it into a bundle. Place the bundle in a fine-mesh sieve suspended over a bowl. Let the "cheese" drain for 4 to 6 hours at room temperature, during which time the microbes from the whey or brine will encourage the probiotic activity in the "cheese." Unmold it from the cheesecloth and chill the cheese for at least 1 hour. Serve chilled or refrigerate it for up to 1 week.

Herbalist Tips

I lean toward using holy basil for medicinal purposes, but culinary basil can also be used for this recipe.

To gather the whey used in this recipe, drain plain, unflavored yogurt in a fine-mesh sieve lined with muslin or cheesecloth over a bowl. The whey collected in the bowl is an excellent source of lactic acid bacteria which promote fermentation. The thickened yogurt can be used as Greek yogurt or drained further for a cream cheese–like consistency. This process can take anywhere from 4 to 12 hours, depending on the desired consistency.

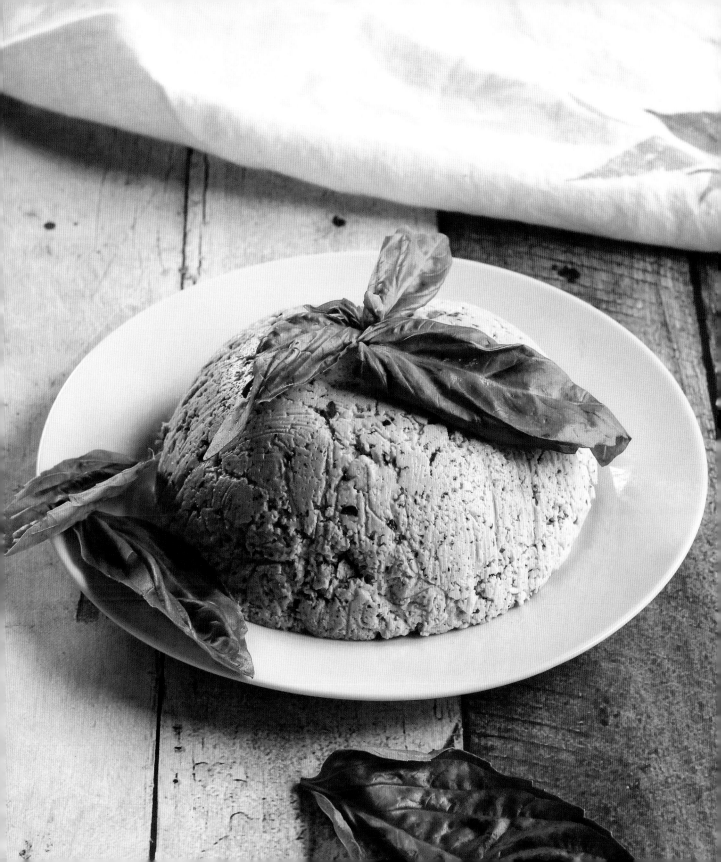

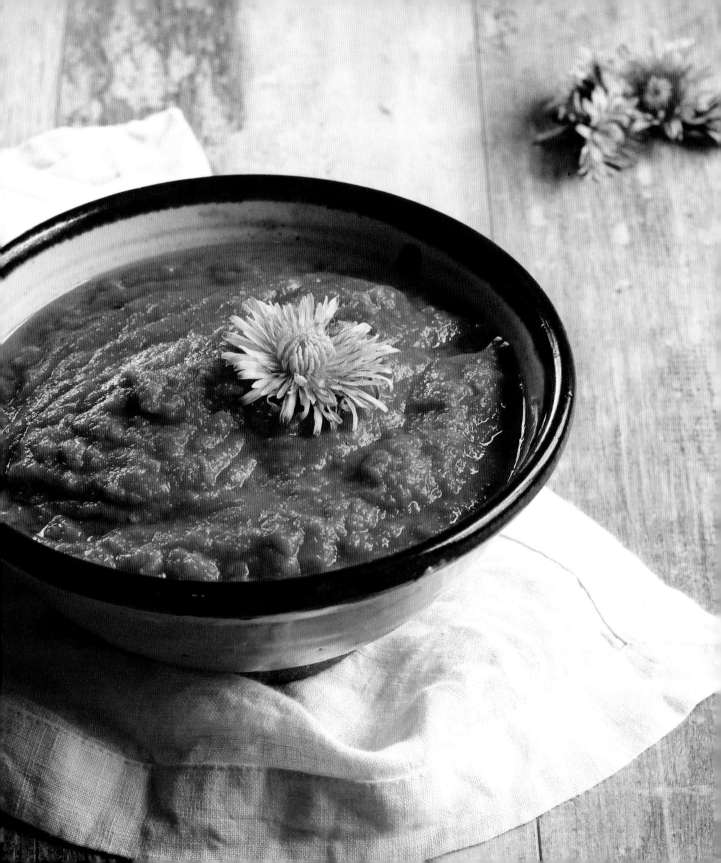

As little kids, many of us often heard: Eat your carrots. They are good for your eyes. The biochemistry involved there is a little more complicated, but carrots are extremely high in a beta-carotenoid known as lutein. Lutein protects eyesight through antioxidant action and supporting the pigmentation and structure of the macula. Dandelion flowers are also a great source of this vital nutrient for eye health. Dried calendula flowers are a nutrient-dense substitute if dandelion flowers are not in season.

This soup is thick, rich and nourishing with roasted flavor and a garlic-y tomato base. An addition of whole-milk Greek yogurt stirred in before serving lends a creamy tang to the soup.

CARROT & DANDELION FLOWER SOUP

Flavor Profile: *Sweet, Pungent*

Serves: *4 to 6*

1½ lb (680 g) carrots, peeled, cut into ½-inch (1.3-cm) slices (about 6 large carrots)

1 large yellow onion, sliced

4–5 cloves garlic, peeled and left whole

2 tbsp (30 ml) extra-virgin olive oil

1 cup (25 g) fresh dandelion blossoms (or ½ cup [15 g] dried dandelion or calendula blossoms)

1 (14.5-oz [411-g]) can whole peeled tomatoes

1 tsp ground cumin

½ cup (100 g) plain Greek yogurt

Salt & freshly ground pepper, to taste

Preheat your oven to 400°F (200°C, or gas mark 6).

Toss the carrots, onion and garlic with olive oil on a rimmed, lined baking sheet. Roast for 20 to 25 minutes, tossing halfway through roasting, until the edges of the vegetables are lightly browned and aromatic.

Meanwhile, bring 2 cups (475 ml) of water to a boil. Pour the water over the dandelion blossoms in a medium-sized bowl. Infuse the water for 20 minutes, then strain it and set aside the "tea" to use in the soup.

Add the roasted vegetables, canned tomatoes, cumin and the dandelion "tea" to a blender or food processor. Blend until it's smooth, about 1 minute. Transfer the mixture to a medium-sized saucepan. Simmer over medium heat for 10 to 15 minutes.

Remove the pan from the heat, and stir in the Greek yogurt. Season with salt and pepper to taste and ladle the soup into bowls.

Deep, rich, saturated colors . . . they are an excellent indicator of the nutrient-load of a food. With very few exceptions, the more naturally vibrant the food, the better it is for you.

Blueberries and spinach promise nutrition with every bite. Blueberries are full of antioxidants, owing to the anthocyanin pigments that give the skins their characteristic blue color. They have been indicated to slow the rate of "mental aging" in humans and increase brain activity associated with intelligence in test animals. Spinach is also high in antioxidants that help to protect the brain and other organs from oxidative stress. Alfalfa, once known as the "king of herbs," is used in this salad as fresh sprouts, lending complex nutrition and texture to this salad.

Sliced almonds add crunch and protein to a simple salad that can be served alongside grilled chicken or tempeh. It is absolutely delicious dressed with the lemon–poppy seed vinaigrette.

BLUEBERRY & SPINACH SALAD WITH LEMON–POPPY SEED VINAIGRETTE

Flavor Profile: *Sour, Sweet, Bitter*
Serves: *4 to 6*

Vinaigrette

¾ cup (175 ml) extra-virgin olive oil

¼ cup (60 ml) fresh lemon juice

1 tbsp (15 g) Dijon mustard

1 tbsp (14 g) mayonnaise

1 tbsp (20 g) raw honey

1 tbsp (9 g) poppy seeds

Salt & freshly ground pepper, to taste

Salad

4 cups (120 g) spinach leaves

1 cup (145 g) fresh blueberries

½ cup (17 g) alfalfa sprouts

½ cup (52 g) sliced almonds

To make the vinaigrette, in a jar with a tight-fitting lid, add the olive oil, lemon juice, mustard, mayonnaise, honey and poppy seeds. Shake the jar vigorously to combine them. Season with salt and pepper to taste.

For the salad, combine the spinach, blueberries, alfalfa sprouts and almonds until they're well combined and evenly distributed. Serve your salad, drizzled lightly with the vinaigrette.

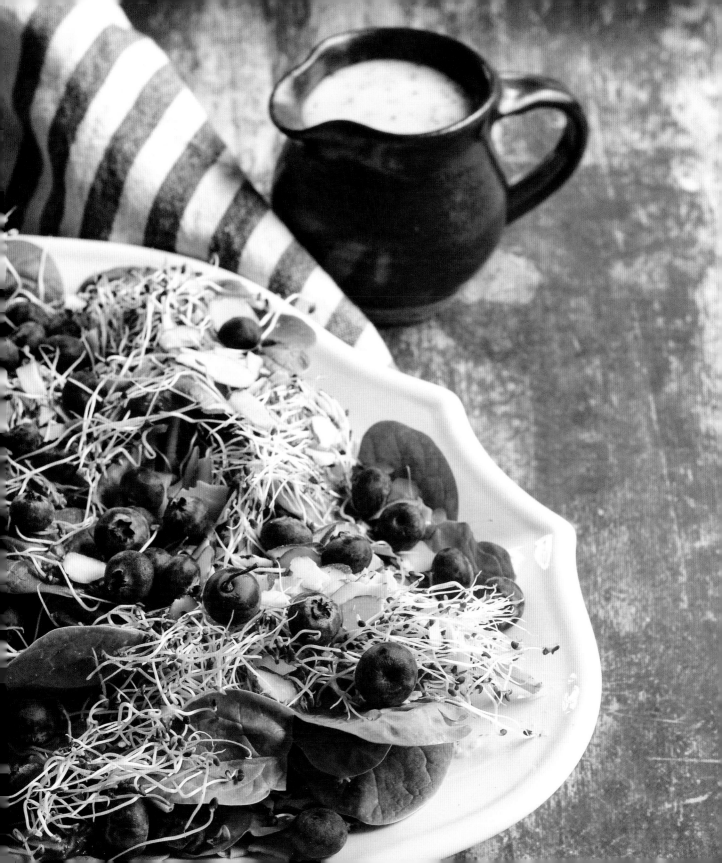

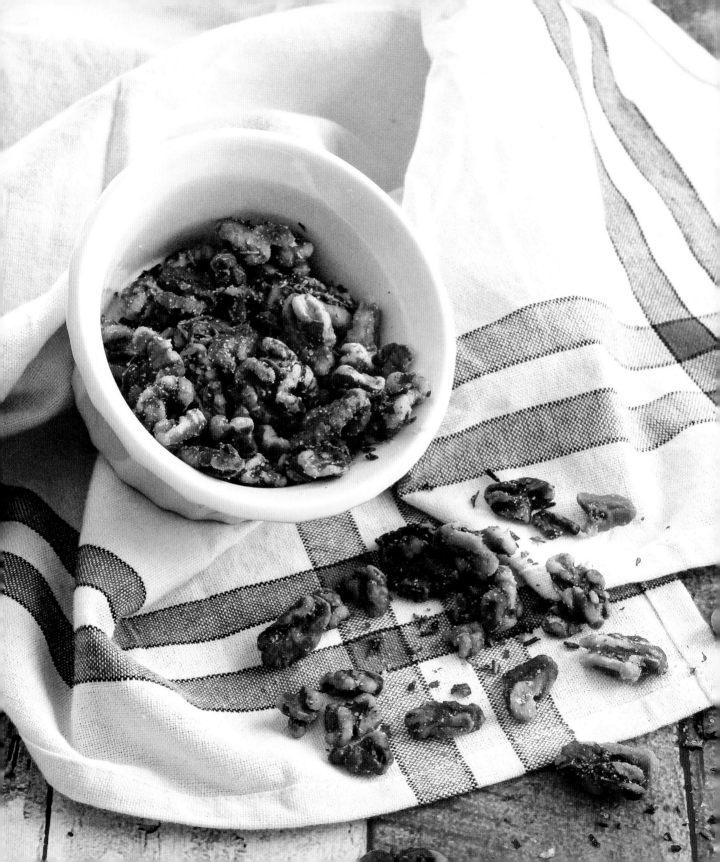

You've probably heard it before: walnuts are brain food and rosemary is for remembrance. Walnuts owe their "brainy" reputation to high levels of omega-3 fatty acids which improve cognition in healthy adults and slow cognitive decline in the elderly population. Heck, if appearance gives us an indication of use, a walnut even resembles a little brain. Rosemary has been indicated as a potent memory enhancer and nourishing stimulant.

This powerhouse duo makes for the perfect afternoon snack, ideal for staving off the post-lunch slump.

ROASTED WALNUTS WITH ROSEMARY

Flavor Profile: *Bitter, Salty*
Makes: *2 cups (200 g)*

2 cups (200 g) raw English walnuts

1 tbsp (15 ml) walnut or olive oil

2 tbsp (4 g) chopped fresh rosemary

½ tsp fine sea salt

Preheat your oven to 325°F (170°C, or gas mark 3). Line a rimmed baking sheet with parchment paper.

In a small bowl, toss the walnuts and oil until the nuts are evenly coated. Place the coated nuts on the lined baking sheet. Roast for 50 to 60 minutes, or until they have a nutty aroma and are very lightly toasted, stirring the nuts occasionally to ensure even browning.

Remove them from the oven and place them in a small bowl. Immediately toss the warm nuts with the rosemary and sea salt. Cool them completely.

Transfer the nuts to a container with an airtight lid and store it in a cool, dry place.

Slipping into the softest clothes you own and sipping a mug of hot chocolate sounds like the ultimate indulgence. But what seems like a purely luxurious act can actually be a bit of self-care. This comforting drink benefits the mind and soul.

Dark chocolate is considered a "brain food" that fuels that epicenter of our being. It is associated with enhanced blood flow to the brain and improved cognitive function in some individuals. Constituents such as theobromine and a small amount of caffeine act as stimulants, offering improved short-term brain function. Add adaptogenic rhodiola root to the mix, and you add mood elevation and increased energy to the picture. Rhodiola imparts a woodsy, floral flavor to this hot chocolate that I find very pleasing.

MINDFUL HOT CHOCOLATE WITH RHODIOLA

Flavor Profile: *Bitter, Sweet*

Serves: *2, generously*

1½ cups (355 ml) whole milk

½ cup (120 ml) half-and-half

2 tsp (10 ml) honey

½ tsp rhodiola root powder

6 oz (170 g) bittersweet chocolate, chopped

Whipped cream, for garnish (optional)

Shaved chocolate, for garnish (optional)

Add the milk, half-and-half, honey, rhodiola root powder and chocolate to a small saucepan. Over medium-low heat, warm the dairy and melt the chocolate. Heat just until it's steaming, but do not simmer, about 3 to 5 minutes.

Ladle the hot chocolate immediately into serving mugs. Top with whipped cream and shaved chocolate, if desired.

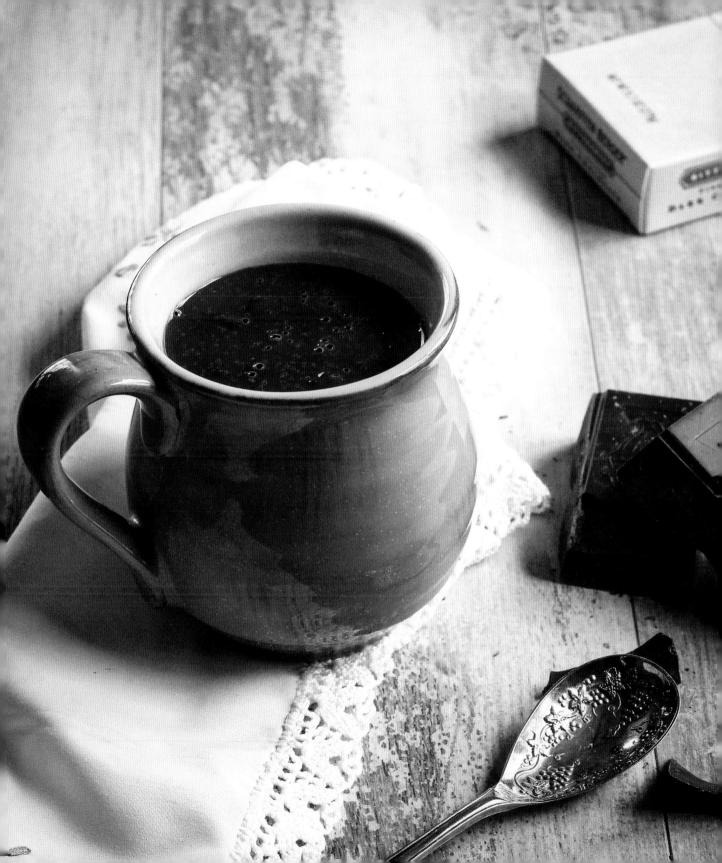

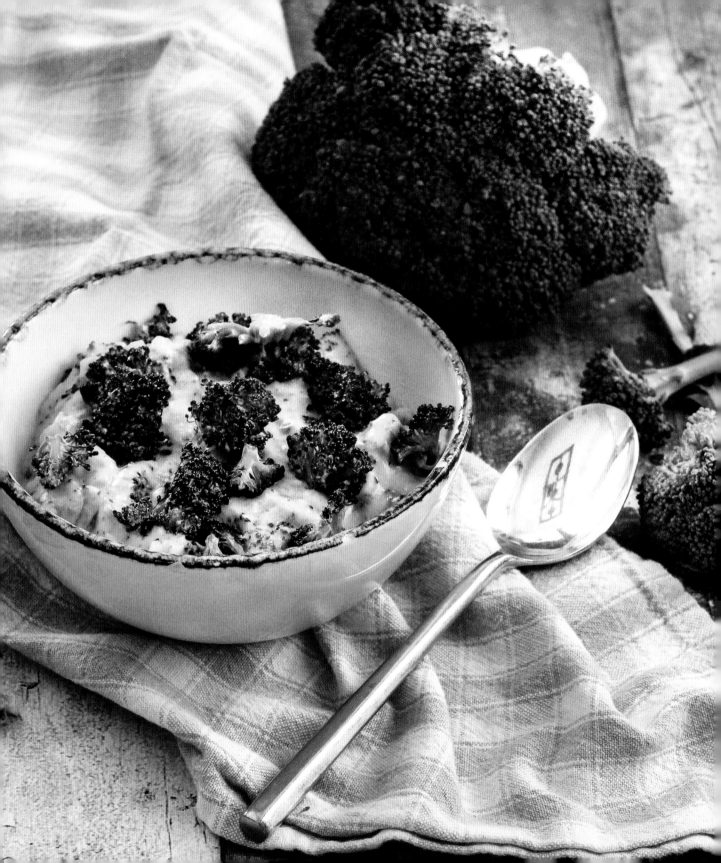

I think broccoli gets an unfair reputation as just another healthy vegetable. It deserves a bit more love and consideration. It is brain food after all!

Broccoli is loaded with vitamins, minerals and phytonutrients that make it a superstar superfood. High in folate and choline, broccoli has the vital nutrients to help maintain cognitive function over time. In this recipe, a small amount of turmeric goes a long way—enhancing the soup's color and adding the neurotrophic benefits of improved cognition and brain function!

Many broccoli and cheddar soup recipes are one dimensional and lack flavor. I change all that by roasting the florets and backing off the cheddar and dairy just enough to give this vegetable its place in the spotlight.

ROASTED BROCCOLI & CHEDDAR SOUP

Flavor Profile: *Bitter, Sweet, Salty*

Serves: *4 to 6*

2 lb (900 g) broccoli, stems sliced and florets broken into bite-size pieces

1 medium-sized yellow onion, diced

2–3 cloves garlic, sliced

2 tbsp (30 ml) extra-virgin olive oil, divided

2 cups (300 g) diced russet potatoes

4 cups (940 ml) Bone Broth with Bone-Building Herbs (page 148) or vegetable broth

1 cup (235 ml) half-and-half

2 tsp (4 g) ground turmeric

1 cup (115 g) shredded cheddar cheese

Salt & freshly ground pepper

Preheat your oven to 400°F (200°C, or gas mark 6).

Toss the broccoli stems, onion and garlic with 1 tablespoon (15 ml) of olive oil in one bowl. Toss the broccoli florets with the other tablespoon (15 ml) of oil in another bowl. Place these on two separate baking sheets and roast until they're lightly golden, about 25 minutes. Remove them from the oven.

In a large stockpot, add the broccoli stems, onion, garlic, potatoes and broth. Bring it to a gentle boil over medium-high heat. Cook until the potatoes are tender, about 15 to 20 minutes. Turn off the heat and puree the soup with an immersion blender until it's smooth. Add the roasted broccoli florets, half-and-half, turmeric and cheddar. Warm the soup over medium heat until it's melted and steamy. Do not boil as this may cause the soup to "break."

Ladle the soup into bowls and serve immediately.

The brain may be the epicenter of our mind and senses, but a complex network of tiny nerves tell our brain about the world around us. Sadly, these nerves can become damaged by injury or disease and can no longer communicate the messages of our senses.

Studies indicate that nerve fibers can be repaired and regenerated with the help of a fascinating and tasty mushroom called lion's mane. While these studies involve highly concentrated extracts, adding lion's mane mushrooms to your diet is another excellent way to support nervous system health. Lion's mane mushroom can be found growing on dead and decaying hardwood logs. They are often grown by specialty mushroom suppliers, and now there are even mushroom growing kits available.

LION'S MANE RISOTTO

Flavor Profile: *Sweet, Salty*

Serves: *4 to 6*

5–6 cups (1.2–1.4 L) mushroom broth

2 cups (340 g) lion's mane mushrooms

1 medium yellow onion, minced

2–3 cloves garlic, minced

3 tbsp (42 g) butter

1¾ cups (350 g) arborio rice or other risotto rice

⅔ cup (160 ml) dry white wine

⅓ cup (28 g) freshly grated Parmesan cheese

2 tbsp (10 g) chopped fresh parsley or chives

Salt & freshly ground pepper, to taste

In a small saucepan, bring the mushroom broth to a gentle simmer over medium-low heat and keep it warm.

In a large saucepan, sauté the mushrooms, onion and garlic in butter over medium heat until the onion is translucent, about 5 minutes. Add the arborio rice. Cook, stirring constantly, for about 2 minutes. Stir in the white wine. As the liquid absorbs, or every 2 to 4 minutes, stir in ½ cup (120 ml) of mushroom broth. Stir frequently. Repeat until the rice is tender, about 25 minutes. Your risotto may require slightly more or less broth than the recipe calls for.

Remove the risotto from the heat and stir in the Parmesan cheese and parsley. Season with salt and pepper to taste. Serve immediately.

Herbalist Tip

To increase the concentration of lion's mane goodness in this recipe, create your own mushroom broth by adding 1 ounce (28 g) of dried lion's mane mushroom powder to 5 to 6 cups (1.2 to 1.4 L) of water. Use this in place of commercial mushroom broth. Lion's mane powder is available from online retailers.

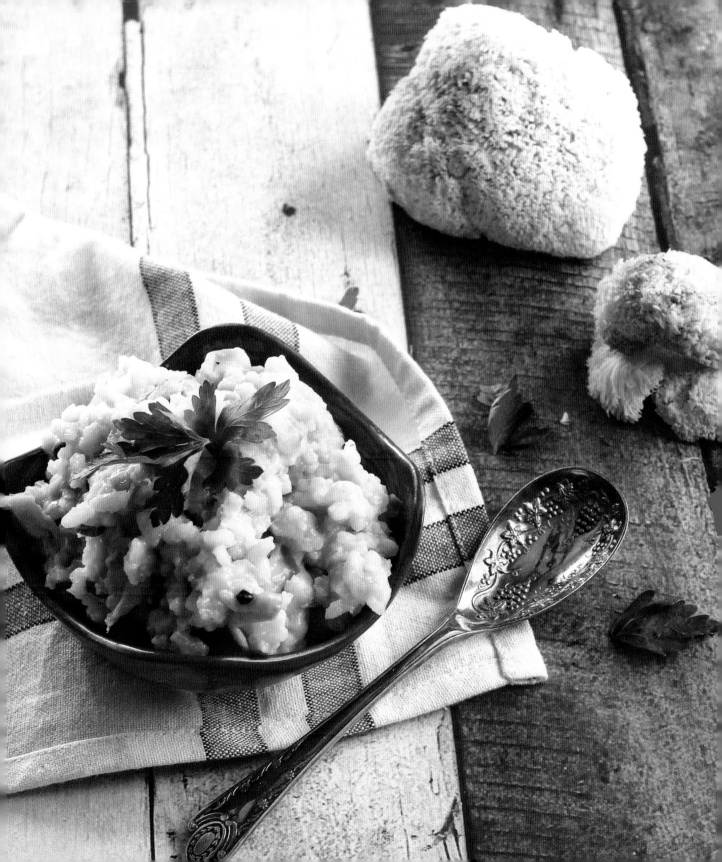

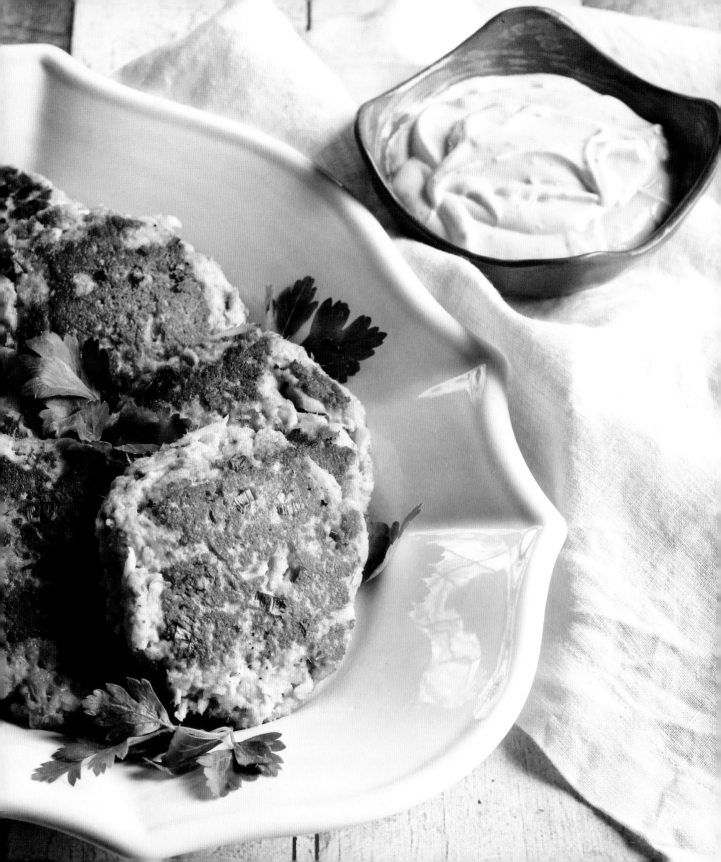

very year my father gives us a case of the most beautiful canned tuna from the local fishermen on the Oregon coast. This ain't no "chicken of the sea." This is the real deal . . . firm, meaty and delicious.

I developed these spicy, flavorful tuna cakes to highlight the ocean's bounty of brain food. Full of omega-3 fatty acids, tuna is fuel for the mind. Studies suggest that frequent consumption of fatty fish, such as salmon and tuna, can slow the rate of age-induced cognitive decline. Delicious Thai basil also acts as an adaptogen, soothing nerves and anxiety, while adding a spicy, clove-like flavor.

Use the best quality canned tuna for this recipe. Please be advised that the current recommendation is to eat no more than 6 ounces (170 g) of tuna per week due to the possibility of high levels of mercury in predatory fish.

ALBACORE TUNA CAKE WITH SRIRACHA AIOLI

Flavor Profile: *Salty, Sweet, Pungent*
Serves: *4*

1 cup (50 g) panko bread crumbs

2 large eggs, lightly beaten

2 cups (280 g) loosely packed albacore tuna

2 tbsp (28 g) mayonnaise

1–2 tsp (5–10 ml) Sriracha or chili sauce

2 scallions, finely minced

2–3 cloves garlic, minced

1 (1-inch [2.5-cm]) piece fresh ginger, grated

Zest of 1 small lemon

2 tbsp (6 g) Thai basil, chopped

1 tsp kosher salt

2 tbsp (30 ml) sesame or peanut oil

Sriracha Aioli

1 cup (225 g) store-bought or homemade mayonnaise

2 tbsp (30 ml) Sriracha or chile paste

Juice of 1 small lemon

In a small bowl, combine the panko, eggs, tuna, mayonnaise, Sriracha, scallions, garlic, ginger, lemon zest, basil and salt. Stir well to combine them. Form eight patties of equal size, about 2½ to 3 inches (6 to 7.5 cm) across and 1 inch (2.5 cm) thick. Chill them on a baking tray in the refrigerator for 30 minutes.

Add the oil to a skillet over medium heat. Cook the patties for 3 to 5 minutes per side, until deep golden brown. Work in batches of three to four patties; do not crowd the pan.

To make the aioli, whisk the mayonnaise, Sriracha and lemon juice well to combine them.

Serve the warm tuna cakes with Sriracha aioli for dipping.

RESOURCES

Desideri, Giovambattista, Catherine Kwik-Uribe, Davide Grassi, Stefano Necozione, Lorenzo Ghiadoni, Daniela Mastroiacovo, Angelo Raffaele, Livia Ferri, Raffaella Bocale, Maria Carmela Lechiara, Carmine Marini and Claudio Ferri. "Benefits in Cognitive Function, Blood Pressure, and Insulin Resistance Through Cocoa Flavanol Consumption in Elderly Subjects with Mild Cognitive Impairment." *Hypertension* 60, no. 3 (2012): 794–801. doi:10.1161/hypertensionaha.112.193060.

Devore, Elizabeth E., Jae Hee Kang, Monique M. B. Breteler and Francine Grodstein. "Dietary Intakes of Berries and Flavonoids in Relation to Cognitive Decline." *Annals of Neurology* 72, no. 1 (2012): 135–43. doi:10.1002/ana.23594.

Essa, Musthafamohamed, Samir Al-Adawi, Mushtaqa Memon, Thamilarasan Manivasagam, Mohammed Akbar and Selvaraju Subash. "Neuroprotective Effects of Berry Fruits on Neurodegenerative Diseases." *Neural Regeneration Research* 9, no. 16 (2014): 1557. doi:10.4103/1673-5374.139483.

Fisher, Naomi D., Meghan Hughes, Marie Gerhard-Herman and Norman K. Hollenberg. "Flavanol-rich Cocoa Induces Nitric-Oxide-Dependent Vasodilation in Healthy Humans." *Journal of Hypertension* 21, no. 12 (2003): 2281–286. doi:10.1097/00004872-200312000-00016.

López, A., T. El-Naggar, M. Dueñas, T. Ortega, I. Estrella, T. Hernández, M.P. Gómez-Serranillos, O.M. Palomino and M.E. Carretero. "Influence of Processing in the Phenolic Composition and Health-Promoting Properties of Lentils (*Lens culinaris* L.)." *Journal of Food Processing and Preservation* 41, no. 5 (2016). doi:10.1111/jfpp.13113.

Lull, Cristina, Harry J. Wichers and Huub F. J. Savelkoul. "Antiinflammatory and Immunomodulating Properties of Fungal Metabolites." *Mediators of Inflammation* 2005, no. 2 (2005): 63–80. doi:10.1155/mi.2005.63.

Mccarty, Mark F., James J. Dinicolantonio and James H. Okeefe. "Capsaicin May Have Important Potential for Promoting Vascular and Metabolic Health." *Open Heart* 2, no. 1 (2015): Table 1. doi:10.1136/openhrt-2015-000262.

Moser, Beate, Thomas Szekeres, Christian Bieglmayer, Karl-Heinz Wagner, Miroslav Mišík, Michael Kundi, Oliwia Zakerska, Armen Nersesyan, Nina Kager, Johann Zahrl, Christine Hoelzl, Veronika Ehrlich and Siegfried Knasmueller. "Impact of Spinach Consumption on DNA Stability in Peripheral Lymphocytes and on Biochemical Blood Parameters: Results of a Human Intervention Trial." *European Journal of Nutrition* 50, no. 7 (2011): 587–94. doi:10.1007/s00394-011-0167-6.

Pianpumepong, Plangpin, Anil Kumar Anal, Galayanee Doungchawee and Athapol Noomhorm. "Study on Enhanced Absorption of Phenolic Compounds of Lactobacillus-fermented Turmeric (*Curcuma longa* Linn.) Beverages in Rats." *International Journal of Food Science & Technology* 47, no. 11 (2012): 2380–87. doi:10.1111/j.1365-2621.2012.03113.x.

Ranasinghe, P., R. Jayawardana, P. Galappaththy, G. R. Constantine, N. De Vas Gunawardana and P. Katulanda. "Efficacy and Safety of 'True' Cinnamon (*Cinnamomum zeylanicum*) as a Pharmaceutical Agent in Diabetes: A Systematic Review and Meta-analysis." *Diabetic Medicine* 29, no. 12 (2012): 1480–492. doi:10.1111/j.1464-5491.2012.03718.x.

Singh, Monika, Talib Hussain, Hina Firdous, Sibhghatulla Shaikh, Syed Mohd Danish Rizvi, Afrasim Moin, Muazzam Khan and Mohammad Amjad Kamal. "Preclinical Hepatoprotective Effect of Herbalism Against Ethanol Induced Hepatotoxicity: A Review." *Current Drug Metabolism* 19, no. 12 (2018): 1002–11. doi:10.2174/1389200219666180330125003.

Smit, Hendrik J., Elizabeth A. Gaffan and Peter J. Rogers. "Methylxanthines Are the Psycho-pharmacologically Active Constituents of Chocolate." *Psychopharmacology* 176, no. 3–4 (2004): 412–19. doi:10.1007/s00213-004-1898-3.

Wong, Kah-Hui, Murali Naidu, Rosie Pamela David, Robiah Bakar and Vikineswary Sabaratnam. "Neuroregenerative Potential of Lions Mane Mushroom, *Hericium erinaceus* (Bull.: Fr.) Pers. (Higher Basidiomycetes), in the Treatment of Peripheral Nerve Injury (Review)." *International Journal of Medicinal Mushrooms* 14, no. 5 (2012): 427–46. doi:10.1615/intjmedmushr.v14.i5.10.

Zare, Roghayeh, Fatemeh Heshmati, Hossein Fallahzadeh and Azadeh Nadjarzadeh. "Effect of Cumin Powder on Body Composition and Lipid Profile in Overweight and Obese Women." *Complementary Therapies in Clinical Practice* 20, no. 4 (2014): 297–301. doi:10.1016/j.ctcp.2014.10.001.

Zhang, Bing, Zeyuan Deng, Yao Tang, Peter X. Chen, Ronghua Liu, D. Dan Ramdath, Qiang Liu, Marta Hernandez and Rong Tsao. Reprint of "Bioaccessibility, In Vitro Antioxidant and Anti-inflammatory Activities of Phenolics in Cooked Green Lentil (*Lens culinaris*)." *Journal of Functional Foods* 38 (2017): 698–705. doi:10.1016/j.jff.2017.03.040.

ACKNOWLEDGMENTS

Thanks to the crew at Page Street Publishing for taking another leap into the complex herbal-wellness world—and for helping me to produce a book as simple as re-seeing the kitchen through the lens of an herbalist. Thank you for having the faith and trust that I could turn the recipes into the remedies.

To my Nitty Gritty Life followers: You guys make all the things possible. Your support is immeasurable.

To my dad, for inviting me into the kitchen and teaching me to cook. To my mom, for teaching me the creativity and resourcefulness to master the arts of homemaking while working. To my extended family, for being so immensely supportive and caring. You have been just the cheering section this writer needs to keep going!

To my wildly creative, inspiring friends in the blogging, writing and wellness world—let's keep bringing health back into the home where it belongs!

To a couple special ladies, Jess & Ivy . . . Ladies, you wipe my tears and tell me to get back on the proverbial horse.

To my children and husband . . . thank you for being my test subjects for the good, the bad and the ugly. I know that all my ferments, wild foods and medicinal meals might make you raise your eyebrows. Thank you for always being willing to try and for offering your honest feedback. Thank you for loving me even when I am unlovable. And thank you for being my home.

ABOUT THE AUTHOR

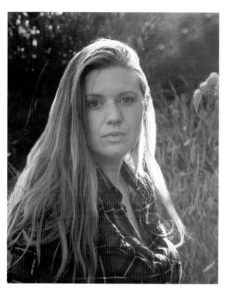

Devon Young homesteads with her husband and children on the westernmost edges of the coastal foothills of the Willamette Valley of Oregon. Renovations continue on their 100-year-old homestead as they reclaim the house and property from the ravages of time and blackberries, and replace it with a warm home and holistic gardens.

Devon has a degree in Complementary and Alternative Medicine from the American College of Healthcare Sciences. She writes about holistic and sustainable living at NittyGrittyLife.com. *The Backyard Herbal Apothecary*, Devon's first book, was published in early 2019. She has written for online resources such as LearningHerbs.com, AttainableSustainable.net and GrowForageCookFerment.com, as well as the *Backwoods Home* magazine.

Devon enjoys foraging, cooking and gardening. She can often be spied trying to balance too many tasks at once, while simultaneously losing her tea.

INDEX